Introduction

This book is particularly useful when used with the A to Z of Peripheral Nerves and, the A to Z of the Bones, Joints, Ligaments & the Back, but all ... to Zs are cross-referenced and together are forming a set ... tural elements of the human body. The A to Z ... muscles, contains the ma... 'ere too numerous to list in ... 'geal muscles involved in slee... first book to cover the br... it is hoped that a book on n... ever increasing series. If there ... see in the A to Zs let us know. Feedback play... A to Zs.

Acknowledgement

Thank you Aspenpharmacare Australia for your support and assistance in this valuable project, particularly Mr. Greg Lan, and Rob Koster. Thank you to all those who have helped when I have been rushed to finish and have made time for this project, and have faith in it, in particular Ante Mihaljevic and Phill Ryman. Thank you everyone who has provided valuable feedback, and help in many ways; Richard, Peter, Robbie, Jody, Quentin, Ximena and there are others too thank you and the namesakes of these books my A to Zs.

Dedication

To all those who have a passion and work hard at it – every day. It all comes down to – you just have to get up in the morning and do it; and then you have to do it again tomorrow.

How to use this book

The structure of the A to Zs grows and develops with each new book while the principle of listing structures in an alphabetical is maintained. Basic anatomical concepts are placed in the beginning of this book; then regional grouping of muscles. The role of the Common Terms section is enlarged, illustrated and colour coded. The text under each muscle in the main listing consists of basic minimal information such as the : Origin (O), Insertion (I), Action (A), Blood Supply (BS), Nerve Supply (NS), Nerve Root origin (NR) and functional tests (T). Naming avoids eponymous terms wherever possible, but if used they are cross referenced with their anatomical name. Capitalization is used to demonstrate the muscles, bones and other important components. The A to Zs may be viewed on 2 sites – www.amandasatoz.com and http://www.aspenpharma.com.au/atlas/student.htm

Thank you

A. L. Neill

BSc MSc MBBS PhD FACBS

ISBN 978-1-921930-188

medicalamanda@gmail

Table of contents

Abbreviations

A = **actions /movements of a joint**
a = artery
aa = anastomosis (ses)
ACF = anterior cranial fossa
adj. = adjective
AKA = also known as
ALL = anterior longitudinal ligament
alt. = alternative
ANS = autonomic nervous system
ant. = anterior
A / P = anterior/posterior
art. = articulation (joint w/o the additional support structures)
AS = Alternative Spelling, generally referring to the diff. b/n UK & USA
assoc. = associated (with)
bc = because
BM = bone marrow
bm = basement membrane
BMD = bone mineral density
b/n = between
br(s) = branch(es)
BS = **blood supply** / blood stream
BV = blood vessel
Bx = biopsy
C = carpal / carpo / cervical
c = cytoplasm
c.f. = compared to
cm = cell membrane
CN = cranial nerve
CNS = central nervous system
Co = collagen
collat. = collateral
CP = cervical plexus
Cr = cranial
CSF = cerebrospinal fluid
CT = connective tissue
D = dermis / diaphysis
DD = differential diagnosis
diff. = difference(s)
DIP = distal interphalangeal joint
dist. = distal
Dx = diagnosis / diagnoses
E = epiphysis
EAM = external acoustic meatus
EC = extracellular (outside the cell)
e.g. = example
EP = epiphyseal growth plate
ER = extensor retinaculum
ES = Erector Spinae group of muscles
er = endoplasmic reticulum
Ex = examination
ext. = extensor (as in muscle to extend across a joint)
ext. = extension
F = fat
f = fluid
FB = fibroblasts
FC = fibrocytes
flex. = flexor
flex. = flexion
FR = flexor retinaculum
gld = gland
GIT = gastro-intestinal tract
Gk. = Greek
grp = group
Histo = Histology
HP = high powered magnification
Hx = history (of the disease)
I = **insertion**
IAS = internal anal sphincter
IC = intercarpal / intercarpo
IMC = intermetacarpal
inf = inferior
IP = interphalangeal
IR = immune response/ reaction

IT = intertarsal
Ix = investigation of
Iy = injury
jt(s) = joints = articulations
l = lymphatic
L = lesion / left / lumbar
lat = lateral
LB = long bone
LBP = low back pain generally assoc with prolapsed disc
LL = lower limb
lig = ligament
longit. = longitudinal
LOF = loss of function
LP = low powered magnification
Lt. = Latin
M = meta
m = muscle
MC = metacarpal / metacarpo
MCF = middle cranial fossa
MCP = metacarpophalangeal
med = medial
mito = mitochondria
MM = mucous membrane
MP = medium magnification
M/P = medial / lateral
MT = metatarsal
mΦ = macrophage
N (s) = nerve(s)
NAD = normal (size, shape)
NAD = no abnormality detected
NK = natural killer
No = nucleolus
NOF = neck of Femur
NR = nerve root origin
NS = nervous supply / nerve system
NT = nervous tissue
Nu = nucleus (nuclei)
nv = neurovascular bundle
O = origin
PAD = peripheral arterial disease
PaNS. = parasympathetic nervous system
ParaNs = parasympathetic nerves ± fibres
partic = particular(ly)
PBM = peak bone mass
PCF = posterior cranial fossa
pH = a measure acidity
ph = phalangeal / phalanges / phalango
PIP = proximal interphalangeal joint
pl. = plural
PLL = posterior longitudinal ligament
PN = peripheral nerve
post. = posterior
proc. = process
prox. = proximal
PS = pubic symphysis
PVD = peripheral vascular disease
Px = progress
R = right / resistance
RA = rheumatoid arthritis
ROM = range of movement
RT = respiratory tract
S = strata/stratum /sacral
SC = spinal cord
SCC = squamous cell carcinoma
sing. = singular
SE = side effects
SN = spinal nerve
SP = spinous process / sacral plexus
SS = signs and symptoms
Su = subcutaneous T / fat
subcut. = subcutaneous (just under the skin) as a site
sup = superior
supf = superficial
SyNS = sympathetic nervous system
T = test / thorax / tissue
TJC = tight junctional complex
TP = transverse process

Tx = treatment / therapy
UL = upper limb, arm
v = very
V = vertebra / vein
VB = vertebral body
VC = vertebral column
vv = vice versa
w = with
WBCs = white blood cells
w/n = within
w/o = without
wrt = with respect to
& = and
∩ = intersection with
= fracture

Common terms in the Study and Examination of Skeletal Muscles, Nerves and Bones

A

Ablation — *(AB-lay-shon)* the removal of part of the body, generally a bony part, most commonly the teeth

Acral — *(AK-ral)* relating to the extremity of an organ or limb –i.e. fingers

Acro — *(AK-roh)-* ***(adj acral) Gk akcron*** **= extreme end, extremity, peak, tip, denoting something at the extremities ankles / fingers / wrists**

Adnexa — *(AD-nex-uh)* appendage, limb extras ***pl adnexae*** *(AD- nex-ee)*

Ala — *(AY-lar)* a wing, hence a wing-like process as in the Ethmoid bone ***pl alae.***

Alveolus — *(AL-vee-oh-lus)* air filled (bone - tooth socket) ***adj alveolar*** (as in air filled bone in the maxilla)

Amorphous — *(AY-mor-fuss)* shapeless, structureless

Anatomical position — the reference position, in which the subject is standing erect with the feet facing forward, arms are at the sides, & the palms of the hands are facing forward (the thumbs are to the outside).

Anatomy — *(ah-NAH-to-mee)* the study of the structure of the body

Ankle — bend = angle usually referring to the bend just above the foot, hence the ankle is the joint b/n the foot & LL

ankylos- — *(an-KEE-los)* **stiff / stiffening – often referring to something becoming calcified**

Ankylosis — **a fixed bending of the jt – unable to straighten – always pathological**

Annulus fibrosis — the peripheral fibrous ring around the intervertebral disc

Aperture — *(a-PET-tyuu-a)* an opening or space b/n bones or w/in a bone.

Aponeurosis — expanded end of a tendon – sheet of fibrous T allowing for muscle insertion

Appendicular — refers to the appendices of the axial i.e. in the skeleton, the limbs upper & lower which hang from the axial skeleton, this also includes the pectoral & pelvic girdles (not the sacrum)

Areola — small, open spaces as in the areolar part of the Maxilla may lead or develop into sinuses.

Arthrodesis — complete loss of movement in a jt due to surgical ablation

Articulation — joint, description of the bone surfaces joining w/o the supporting structures = point of contact b/n 2

	opposing bones hence the articulation of Humerus & Scapula is the articulation of the shoulder joint. ***adj articular***
Artifact	*(AH-te-fact)* AS **Artefact** – any distortion seen in the histological or radiological processing of material
Atopy	*(AY-toe-pee)* – out of place ***adj atopic***
Auditory	pertaining to hearing, hence, pertaining to the ear.
Axial	*(AK-see-el)* refers to the head & trunk (vertebrae, ribs & sternum) of the body as opposed to appendicular.

B

Ball and Socket	generally referring to a joint which resembles a ball sitting tightly in a socket - very stable, limited range of movement e.g. hip joint
Basement membrane (bm)	a thin layer of extracellular fibrillar protein matrix & CT stroma that underlies all epithelial cells
baso-	base (as in acid / base; as in the bottom – the basal layer) ***adj basal***
Basocranium	bones of the base of the skull
-blast	immature cell / undifferentiated cell
Bone	*(BOH-n)* a CT that contains a hardened matrix of mineral salts & collagen fibers. Bone cells include: osteoblasts, osteocytes, & osteoclasts.
Boss	a smooth round broad eminence - mainly in the frontal bone ♀ > ♂
Brachial	*(BRAY kee-al)* arm, mainly to do with the upper arm
Bregma	refers to a junction of more than 2 bones in a jt as in the Bregma of the skull, junction b/n the coronal & sagittal sutures which in the infant is not closed & can be felt pulsating
Brevis	short
Buccal	pertaining to the cheek
Bursa	*(BER-suh)* a flattened sac containing a film of fluid (B), found around jts to allow for movement. **pl bursae** e.g. the Elbow jt bursa. b/n Humerus (H) & Ulna (U)

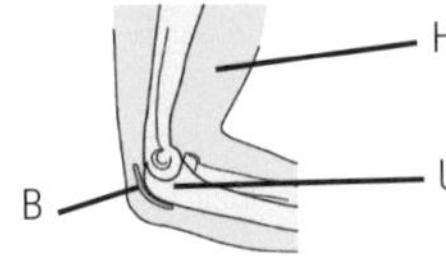

C

Calcaneus — *(KAL-kan-ee-us)* heel, hence the bone of the heel ***adj calcaneal.***

Calcaneal tendon — ***see Achilles tendon***

Calcar — a spur ***adj calcarine.***

Calcinosis — *(KAL-sin-oh-sis)* deposits of Calcium in body Ts &/or organs

Calotte — *(KALoh-tee)* the Calotte consists of the Calvaria from which the base has been removed.

Calvaria — the Calvaria are the bones of the Cranium w/o the facial bones, attached.

Camptodactyly — congenital flexion disorder of the PIP, generally affects the little finger

Canal — tunnel / extended foramen as in the carotid canal at the base of the skull ***adj canular***

Canaliculus — small canal

Cancellous bone — **= Trabecular bone** a spongy, porous bone, lightweight with bone spicules or trabeculae parallel to lines of force found at the ends of LBs (epiphyses) with surrounding BM, found sandwiched b/n lamellae of compact bone, in the VBs & in areas of ⬆ bone thickness

Cancer — *(KAN –ser)* group of diseases where the cells w/o the normal controls

Capitulum — diminutive of Caput, little head

Capsule — *(KAP-syoo-l)* an enclosing membrane

Caput / Kaput — the head or of a head, ***adj.- capitate = having a head (c.f. decapitate)***

Carpal Tunnel — the tunnel formed by the wrist bones (carpal bones) to allow the passage of the flexor tendons & Ns to the hand & fingers , bound superiorly by the palmar fascia

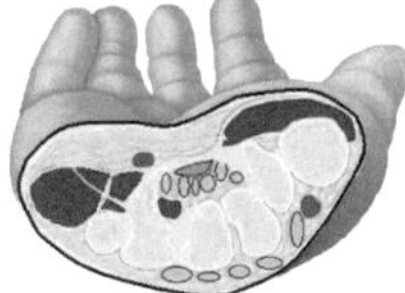

Carpo — wrist

Carpometacarpal — generally referring to the jt b/n hand & the wrist bones

Cartilage — *(KAR-tih-lehj)* a type of CT characterized by the presence of an extensive matrix containing a dense distribution of proteins & a thickened GS.

Cavity *(KAV-it-ee)* an open area or sinus w/in a bone or formed by 2 or more bones ***adj cavernous***, may be used interchangeably with fossa. Cavity tends to be more enclosed fossa a shallower bowl-like space (e.g. Orbital fossa-Orbital cavity).

Cavum a cave ***adj cavis***

Cell *(SELL)* the basic living unit of multicellular organisms.

Cephalic pertaining to the head

Cervico- pertaining to the neck

chondro- *(KON-droh)* referring to cartilage

Chondrium *(KON-dree- um)* the cartilage ***adj chondria, chondral***

Chondrocyte *(KON-droh-site)* a mature cartilage cell.

Chondroitin sulphate *(kon-DROI-tin SUL-fate)* a semisolid material forming part of the EC matrix in certain CT.

chromo- *(KROHM-oh)* referring to colour ***adj chromatic***

Cillia pertaining to eyelash and hair

Clavicle little key = S-shaped bone = collar bone

Cochlea *(KOK-lee-uh)* a snail hence snail-like shape relating to the Organ of Corti

Collagen *(KOL-a-jen)* the major fibre of the body; in CT, tendons ligaments & extracellular substances of many Ts

Colle's referring to a collar or neck

Compact bone **= Cortical bone = Dense bone** bone found in the shafts & on external bone surfaces. The structure is variable & constantly being remodeled throughout life. It may consist of osteons &/or lamellae.

Concha *(KON-kuh)* a shell shaped bone as in the ear or nose ***(pl. conchae adj. chonchoid)*** old term for this turbinate.

Condyle *(KON-dial)* a rounded enlargement or process – used in ref to a number of bones – commonly the TMJ jt

Congenital *(KON-jen-it-al)* present from birth

Connective tissue *(kon-EK-tiv Tish-ew)* (CT) one of the 4 basic types of tissue in the body. It is characterized by an abundance of EC material with relatively few cells & functions in the support & binding of body structures.

Cornu a horn (as in the Hyoid)

Corona a crown. ***adj coronary, coronoid or coronal;*** hence a coronal plane is parallel to the main arch of a crown which passes from ear to ear ***(c.f. coronal suture).***

Cortex the rind or the bark of the tree
Costo/Costa - pertaining to the ribs
Coxa hip
Cranium the cranium of the skull comprises all of the bones of the skull except for the mandible.
Crest prominent sharp thin ridge of bone formed by the attachment of muscles particularly powerful ones e.g. Temporalis/Sagittal crest
Cribiform / Ethmoid a sieve or bone with small sieve-like holes.
Crown = Vertex the top of the organ or body
Crura ***adj cruris*** leg
Cuneate /Cuneus a wedge / wedge-shaped (bone)
cyst- (SIST) **bladder / fluid filled sac**
-cytes (SYTS) **mature cell types**
cyto- **cellular**

D

dactyly **digits**
dendro- tree-like formation
Deltoid D-shaped
Dens a tooth hence dentine & dental relating to teeth, denticulate having tooth-like projections ***adj dentate see also odontoid***
Depression a concavity on a surface
Dermatome section of skin (3) supplied by a single NR (2) as opposed to myotome (1) – which is the area of muscle supplied by a single NR – skin & muscle supplied by the same NR are generally closely associated

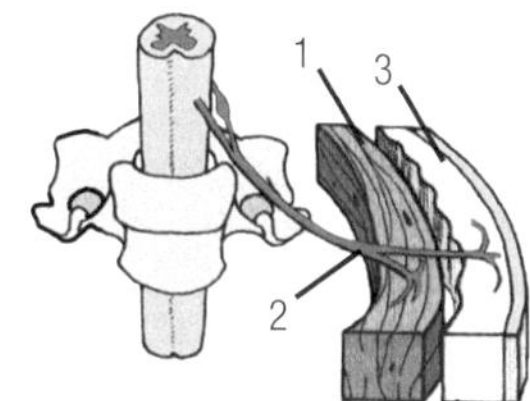

Diaphragm a partition or separating wall
Diaphysis *(DY-af-i-sis)* the shaft or body of a LB. In the young this is the region b/n the growth plates & is composed of compact bone. ***pl = diaphyses adj = diaphyseal***
Diarthrodal jt **= synovial jt = moveable jt**

Diastasis separation – may mean separation of a muscle from its original position as in pregnancy; or a bone from its original position w/o # – as in tendon rupture

Differentiation the changing of cells to become increasingly specialized

Digit / Digitorum relating to fingers and toes

Diploë the cancellous bone b/n the inner & outer tables of the skull, ***adj diploic.***

Dislocation a displacement of anything e.g. a joint

Distal further away from the axial skeleton *(opposite of Proximal)*

dorsi- back

dys- *(DIS)* ***Gk bad sign*** **abnormal, bad, difficult, disorganized, painful (opposite to eu)**

Dysplasia *(DIS-play-zee-yah)* abnormal growth of T or cells

E

Edentulous w/o teeth

Effusion excess synovial fluid – in the jt

Elbow any angular bend, e.g.in the UL, referring to the jt b/n the arm & forearm

Eminence a smooth projection or elevation on a bone as in iliopubic eminence.

Endocranium refers to the interior of the "braincase" ***adj. endocranial*** divided into the 3 major fossae anterior (for the Frontal lobes) middle (containing Temporal lobes) and posterior (for the containment of the Cerebellum).

Endogenous growing from w/in tissues or cells

Endostium a mesodermal CT which lines the inner surface of all bones & is the conduit for the NS & BS of the bone. Lifting of the endosteum causes cancellous bone to be laid down to fill the gap b/n the bone & the cellular layer & this device may be used to encourage bone growth/repair.

Enostosis = bony island a bony growth of compact bone w/in a bone – generally on the internal surface in the trabecular bone harmless incidental finding – DD prostatic metastasis

epi- **on top of**

Epiphysis the end of a LB beyond the growth plate or EP. Generally develops as a 20 ossification centre. There are 2 epiphyses to each LB. Of a LB the shafts are generally compact bone & the ends = epiphyses are trabecular bone with a compact bone covering ***pl.= epiphyses adj.= epiphyseal***

Excrescence outgrowth from a surface – e.g. normal fingernail / abnormal wart or exostosis

Exostosis a bony outgrowth from a bony surface, often due to irritation (as in Swimmer's ear) & may involve ossification of surrounding Ts such as muscles or ligaments.

F

Facet a face, a small bony surface (occlusal facet on the chewing surfaces of the teeth) seen in planar joints.

Falciform *(FAL-see form)* relating to shapes that are in a sickle shape so falciform ligaments curve around & end in a sharp point

Fascia *(FASH-ee-ah)* ***Lt = a band*** a sheet or band of fibrous T deep in the skin covering & attaching to deeper tissues

Fascicle *(FAS-ih-kul)* small bundle

Femoral angle the angle b/n the femoral head & the shaft normal 120º - 135º, Valgus >135º, Varus < 120º

Fibroblast an immature progenitor cell found in all CT, capable of mitosis, migration, movement. Among other pathways they develop into fibrocytes.

Fibrocyte **mature fibre producing cell = mature fibroblast – ** spindle shaped cell producing either collagen (col) or elastin (e) fibres via secretion of monomer units (m) which assemble outside the cell into long fibres, which are then maintained by the fibrocytes. Note with age the number of fibrocytes & hence the fibres ⬇ hence compromising the integrity & strength of their CT.

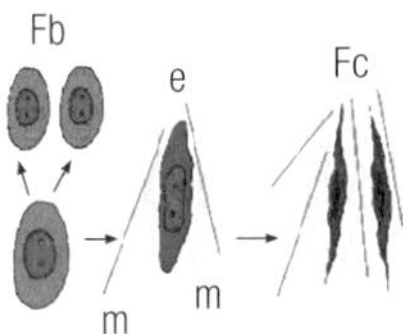

Fibrocartilagenous stroma background T of cartilage with high collagen fibre component

Fibromatosis fibrosis w/n a fascial sheath

Fibrosis *(FY- broh-sis)* ⬆ fibrous T, generally collagen fibres as in scars; can occur in all organs

Fissure a narrow slit or gap from cleft.

Foramen a natural hole in a bone usually for the transmission of BVs &/or Ns. ***pl. foramina.***

Fornix an arch

Fossa a pit, depression, or concavity, on a bone, or formed from several bones as in temporomandibular fossa. Shallower & more like a "bowl" than a cavity

Fovea a small pit (usually smaller than a fossa) - as in the fovea of the occlusal surface of the molar tooth.

Fracture (#) a break, generally referring to bone

Fusiform spindle-shaped – many CT cells are of this shape particularly fibrocytes.

G

Geneio referring to the chin

Genu *(JEN-you)* knee ***adj genio*** referring to the knee

Genu Recurvatum – hyperextension of the knee jt

Genu Valgus – knock-kneed **("G" knocking together)**

Genu Varus – bow-legged **(AR – AIR in b/n)**

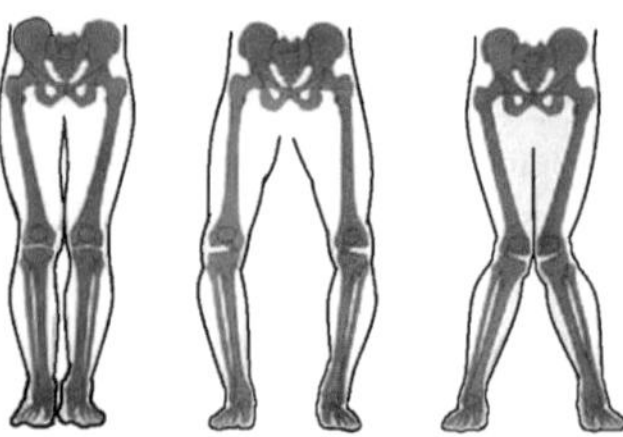

Genu Norma Genu Varus Genu Valgus

Glossus referring to the tongue

Gluteal referring to the buttocks

Groove a long pit or furrow as on the Humerus – may be due to muscle tracking

H

haemo *(HEEM-oh)* **AS hemo- referring to blood**

Hallux the big toe = the first toe

Hamus a hook hence the term used for bones which "hook around other bones or where other structures are able to attach by hooking - hamulus = a small hook.

Harris lines **AKA growth arrest lines** lines of ⬆ bone density due to pathological assault or sudden growth spurts. They indicate the position of the EP at the time of the event but they may change the shape of the bone & affect its length. Only seen in Xrays

Haversian canals **= osteons *see Osteons***

Hinge joint jt with movement in one plane e.g. elbow or knee

Hormone ***Gk hormaein = to spur on*** a substance secreted in the body having a regulatory affect on organs & Ts

Hyoid U-shaped

Hyperostosis abnormal bone growth, thickening, generally overgrowth or ectopic growth

hypo- **underneath / below**

I

Ideopathic of unknown origin

Incisura a notch

Inclusion any foreign or heterogeneous substance w/in a cell not introduced as a result of trauma.

Inferior under

Inter between

Intra within

Intracellular inside the cell

Introitus *(In-TROY-tus)* an orifice or point of entry to a cavity or space.

J

Joint **= Articulation + supporting structures**

L

Lacerum something lacerated, mangled or torn e.g. foramen lacerum small sharp hole at the base of the skull - often ripping T in trauma.

Lacrimal related to tears & tear drops. ***(noun lacrima)***

Lambda ***Gk letter a capital 'L'*** - written as an inverted V. ***adj lambdoid*** – used to name the point of connection b/n 3 skull bones Occipital and L & R Temporal bones.

Lamina a plate as in the lamina of the vertebra a plate of bone connecting the vertical & transverse spines ***(adj lamellar, pl. laminae) e.g. lamellar bone*** layers of compact bone interdigitated with sheets

	of collagen fibres these may form concentric rings around BVs as in osteons (Haversian systems) or as layers around the outside & inside of the diaphysis of LBs
Lamina dura	layer of immature bone lining the tooth socket
Lesion	any single area of altered tissue or part of an organ
leuco-/ leuko-	**AKA luco /luko** *(LOO- koh)* white, pale, clear
Leucocyte	***see white blood cell (WBC)***
Ligament (s)	a band of CT which connects bones (articular ligaments) (1) or viscera - organs (visceral ligaments), generally collagen A ligament is a tie or a connection. Originally it was used as sing. ***ligamentum pl ligamenta*** from ligate or to tie up generally composed of collagen fibres. ***see also Tendons*** (2)

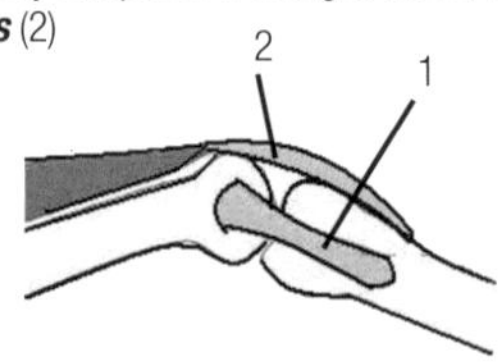

Linea	a line as in the Nuchal lines of the Occipitum / Occipital bone
Lingus	*(ling-GUS)* tongue ***adj Lingual*** *(ling-GEW-al)* pertaining to the tongue
Lip	projection over the usual marging
Lipping	bone projecting over the usual margin, excessive production generally pathological as in OA, may interfere with jt movement
Locus	*(LOH-kus)* a place ***(c.f. location, locate, dislocate)*** – specific area in organ or T of either cell division or specialization
Lordosis	*(lor-DOH-sis)* concavity in the VC – cervical & lumbar region have this normal curve which may become exaggerated – predisposes to LBP ***opposite to kyphosis***
-lucent	*(LOO-sent)* transparent, clear
-lymph	*(LIM-pf)* clear liquid
Lumbar	back – generally the lower back as in **Lumbago**
Lymphatic	a vessel which carries fluid – lymph - to the heart
Lysosomes	toxic cellular organelles containing enzymes which digest material – if lysed they will destroy their host cell

M

macro- **big, large**

Magnum large ***pl magna***

Malleus hammer (as in the ear ossicle)

Mandible from the verb to chew, hence, the movable lower jaw; ***adj mandibular.***

Mastoid breast or teat shape - mastoid process of the Temporal bone.

Maxilla the jaw-bone; now used only for the upper jaw; ***adj maxillary.***

Meatus a short passage; ***adj meatal*** as in EAM connecting the outer ear with the middle ear.

Meniscus ***Gk. crescent*** – relating to the cartilaginous intra-articular crescents in the knee jt

Mentum relating to the chin (mentum = chin not mens = mind) ***adj mental.***

Meta an extension of…: cf. metacarpal = extension of the wrist

Metacarpophalangeal (MCP AKA MP) generally referring to the jt b/n hand & finger

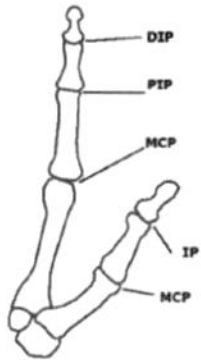

DIP
PIP
MCP
IP
MCP

Metaphysis **= Epiphysis** the slightly expanded end of the shaft of a bone.

Metaplasia the changing of one form of T type to another, extending from one type to another type as it grows

Micronutrient similar to trace element but it includes any substance which is essential to the body's normal functioning but is only needed in minute amounts. Deficiencies are rare in most cases because the dietary needs are so low; they often involve bone metabolism. Common micronutrients are: Aluminum, Boron, Chromium, Copper, Fluoride, Manganese, Molybdenum, Silicon, Zinc

morph- *(MORF-)* **shape / form**

Mucus *(MEW-kus)* slippery gelatinous substance produced by mucoid glands AKA phlegm ***adj mucous also mucoid*** **– mucus-like & myxoid** *(MIKS-oyd)* generally referring to substances found in Tms which have a mucus-like appearance slimy & jelly – in these cases it is pathological

Multiforme — ***see also Polymorphic***

myco- — *(MY-coh)* **relating to fungi**

myelo- — *(MY-loh)* **to do with the BM or the SC**

Myotome — section of muscle (1) supplied by a single NR (2) as opposed to dermatome (3) – which is the area of skin supplied by a single NR – skin & muscle supplied by the same NR are generally closely associated

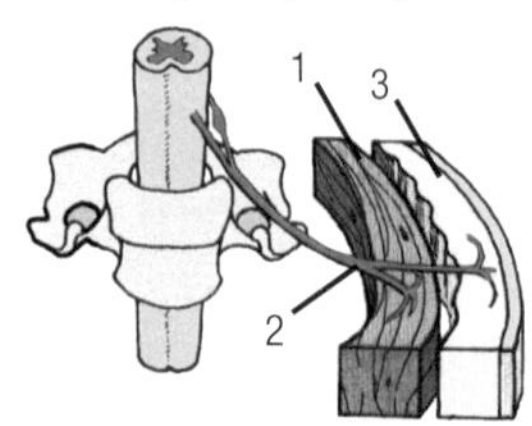

N

Neurocranium — the neurocranium refers only to the braincase of the skull.

Neuroma — benign proliferation of neural T but is often used to denote a fibrosis / fibrous nodule particularly in the feet as in plantar neuroma

noci- — *(NOH-see)* **pain**

Notch — an indentation in the margin of a structure.

Nucha — *(NEW-kuh)* the nape or back of the neck ***adj nuchal***

Nucleus — *(NEW-klee-us)* nut – brain of the cell containing DNA
Nucleolus *(NEW-klee OH-lus)*
brain w/n the brain - nub of DNA material inside the nucleus

O

Occiput — the prominent convexity of the back of the head
Occipitum = Occipital bone ***adj. occipital***

occulta — hidden

Occulus — an eye

Odontoid — relating to teeth, tooth like ***see Dens***

Oedema — **AS Edema** *(uh-DEEM-uh)* swollen ***adj oedematous***

-oid — **like / similar to**

-ology — **study of**

-oma — **lump / tumour**

Omo — *(OH-moh)* shoulder

Ontogeny — the development of an individual growth pattern

Orbit a circle; the name given to the bony socket in which the eyeball rotates; ***adj orbital.***

Organelles small intracellular structures e.g. mitochondria

Orifice an opening.

ortho- **straight**

Orthosis **AKA orthotic device** device to correct the movement of a bone or bones – from the simple foot orthoses to complex neck braces - the study of which device to use or make is the study of orthotics ***pl orthoses***

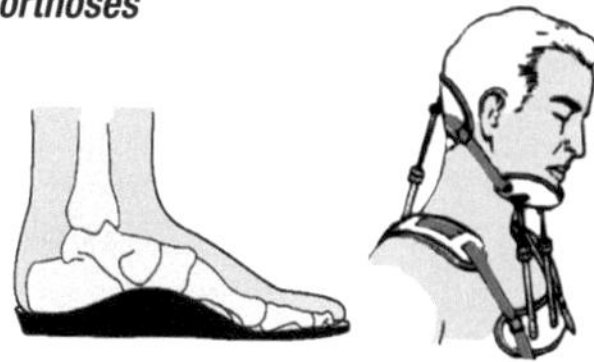

Orthosis general bone disease

Os a bone or pertaining to bones ***adj osseus***

-osis **disease of – non-inflammatory – implying a degeneration**

Ossicle a small bone as in the ear ossicles: Stapes (stirrup), Incus (anvil) & Malleus (hammer).

Ossification the process of turning something into bone, i.e. from one T to another as in cartilaginous ossification from cartilage into bone Two other forms are 1° ossification (in the shaft of the LB where the bone forms from CT) & 2° ossification where the bone has formed & 2° centers develop as at the ends of the LBs).

Ostium *(o-STEE-um)* a door, an opening, an orifice.

Otic pertaining to the ear

Ovale oval shaped

P

Palate a roof ***adj palatal or palatine.***

para- ***Gk* to one side**

Paratendinitis If changes w/n the tendon sheath

Parietal pertaining to the outer wall of a cavity; from paries = a wall.

Parotid pertaining to a region beside or near the ear

Pars a part of

Patella kneecap

-pathy **disease of**
Pedis *(PED-is)* pertaining to feet
-penia *(PEEN-ee-yuh)* lack of
peri- around
Perikymata transverse ridges & the grooves on the surfaces of teeth
Perivascular surrounding BVs generally capillaries
Periosteum layer of fascial tissue CT on the outside of compact bone not present on articular (joint) surfaces ***see endosteum***
Periostitis inflammation on the outer surface of the bone
Periostosis abnormal growth of LBs on their outer surfaces
Pes any part of the LL below the ankle – generally refers to the foot
Petrous pertaining to a rock / rocky / stony ***adj petrosal***
phaeo- *(FAY-oh)* **brown dusky**
phago *(FAY-goh)* **to eat / eater**
Phalanx pertaining to flanks of soldiers - phalanges a row of soldiers used for a row of fingers or toes ***adj phalangeal as in interphalangeal jts see metacarophalangeal jts***
-phil *(FILL)* **lover of**
-phobe *(FOBE)* **hater of**
Planar joints jt which allows for sliding across the jt as in the wrist, foot & ribs
-plasia *(PLAY-see-yu)* **growth**
-pluri- **multiple**
-podia formation *(POH-dee-yu)* **pertaining to feet (often the of feet for cell movement)**
poikilo- *(POYK-il-oh)* **spotted, mottled, irregular**
poly- **many**
Polymorphic many shaped ***see also Multiforme***
Pollex thumb
Process a general term describing any marked projection or prominence as in the mandibular process.
Prominens a projection
Proximal closer to the axial skeleton (opposite of distal)
pseudo *(SEW-doh)* **false**
Pterion *(TERY-on)* a wing; the region where the tip of the greater wing of the sphenoid meets or is close to the parietal, separating the frontal from the squamous region of the Temporal bone ***adj pterygoid.***
Pubis hairy – that part of the hip bone with hair over the surface ***adj pubic pl pubes***

R

Rachitic *(RAK-it-ik)* description of the uncalcified osteochondroid mixture observed in rickets – & Vitamin D deficiencies

Ramus branch as in the superior pubic ramus the superior or higher branch of the pubic bone (Pubis)

Recess a secluded area or pocket; a small cavity set apart from a main cavity.

Rectus *(REK-tus)* **AKA ortho** straight – erect

recte- **straight** ***adj recticular***

Reduction the return of a bone or joint to its proper place after dislocation &/or subluxation

Re-modeling the forming & reforming of bone in its normal growth cycle

Rotundum round

S

Sagittal an arrow, the sagittal suture is notched posteriorly, making it look like an arrow by the lambdoid sutures.

Salpingo pertaining to a tube

Scalene uneven

Sclerosis hard / hardening ***adj sclerotic***

Sella a saddle; ***adj sellar,*** sella turcica = Turkish saddle.

Sesamoid grainlike

Sigmoid S-shaped, from the letter Sigma which is S in Greek.

Skull the skull refers to all of the bones that comprise the head.

Spheno *(SFVEE-noh)* a wedge i.e. the Sphenoid is the bone which wedges in the base of the skull b/n the unpaired Frontal & Occipital bones ***adj sphenoid.***

Spine a thorn ***adj spinous*** descriptive of a sharp, slender process / protrusion.

Splanchocranium the facial bones of the skull.

spondy- **to do with the vertebra, or vertebral column**

Squamous flat, square-shaped

Stroma background T which may be fibrillar with occasional resident cells present, or matrix & extracellular material, in a T, GS & the assoc. cells present which do not represent the main T or organ

Subchondral beneath cartilage – generally referring to the bone just below the articular cartilage

Subluxation minor dislocation

Sulcus long wide groove often due to a BV indentation

Supine to place face up ***(opp Prone)***

Sustenaculum a supportive structure as in the sustenaculum tali = a structure which supports the Talus in the foot

Suture the saw-like edge of a cranial bone that serves as jt b/n bones of the skull.

Stylos an instrument for writing hence ***adj styloid*** a pencil-like structure.

Symphysis a cartilagenous joint or a growth with bone-cartilage-bone

syn- **means together i.e. the close proximity of, or fusion of 2 structures**

Syndesmosis tight inflexible joints b/n 2 bones little to no movement as in many axial joints

Synostosis fusion of any joints

Synovial joint **= Diarthrosis** any moveable joint with synovial fluid b/n the 2 opposing bones – most moving joints are synovial.

Systemic *(SIS-tem-ik)* involving the whole body

T

Talus *(TAY-lus)* ankle ***(Gk. bend)***

Tarsus pertaining to any bones joining the foot with the leg ***adj tarsal (Gk wickerwork referring to the basket like structure of the os tarsus with the ligaments)***

- taxis **locomotor movement of cells**

Tectum a roof.

Tegmen a covering.

Temporal refers to time & the fact that grey hair (marking the passage of time) often appears first at the site of the Temporalis.

Tendo Calcaneus anatomical name for Achilles tendon – ***see also Calcaneal tendon***

Tendon a tie or cord of collagen fibres connecting muscle with bone (as opposed to articular ligaments which connect bone with bone)

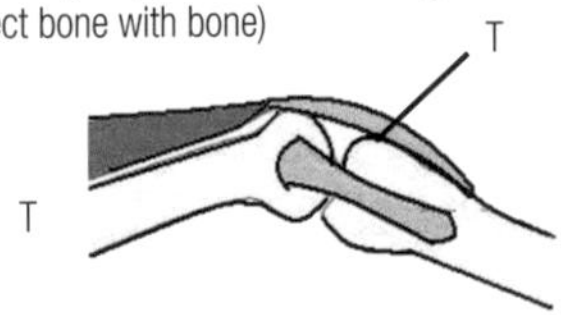

T

T

Tentorium a tent.

Tibiofemoral angle ***see also Q angle*** the angle b/n the Femoral shaft & the Tibia

Trabecula a "little" beam i.e. supporting structure or strut ***pl trabeculae***

Trochanter pertaining to a small wheel or disc in the Femur it is a large disc shaped tuberosity

Trochlea a pulley, that part of the bone or ligamentous attachment that pulls the bone in another direction as in the elbow or the ankle

Tubercle a small process or bump, an eminence.

Tuberculum a very small prominence, process or bump.

Tuberosity a large rounded process or eminence, a swelling or large rough prominence often associated with a tendon or ligament attachment.

U

Uncus a hook ***adj uncinate.***

V

Vertex top, superior point

Volkmann's canal **= perforating canal** connecting channels in compact bone b/n osteons & perforating the lamellae of the osteon & bringing in the periosteal lining

Volvar pertaining to the sole of the foot or palm of hand

W

White blood cells **(WBC) = leucocytes** general term for all blood borne cells which appear white on the blood smear / BM smear – includes: monocytes, lymphocytes & granulocytes

Wormian bone extrasutural bone in the skull

Z

Zygoma a yoke, hence, the bone joining the Frontal, Maxillary, Sphenoid & Temporal bones ***adj zygomatic.***

Structure and Substructure of Skeletal muscles

1 muscle *eg. Biceps*
2 epimysium - CT *surrounding a whole muscle*
3 perimysium - CT *surrounding a muscle fascicle*
4 endomysium - CT *surrounding each muscle fibre*
5 muscle fibre
6 nucleus *(note the muscle cell is multinucleated)*
7 sarcolemma - membrane *around each myofibril*
8 myofibril
9 sarcomere *basic contractile unit of the muscle*
10 myosin filament
11 actin filament

A band - myosin to myosin filaments
H band - myosin only segments *minimum in contraction*
I band - actin only segment maximum in relaxation
Z line - line of attachment of the actin filaments

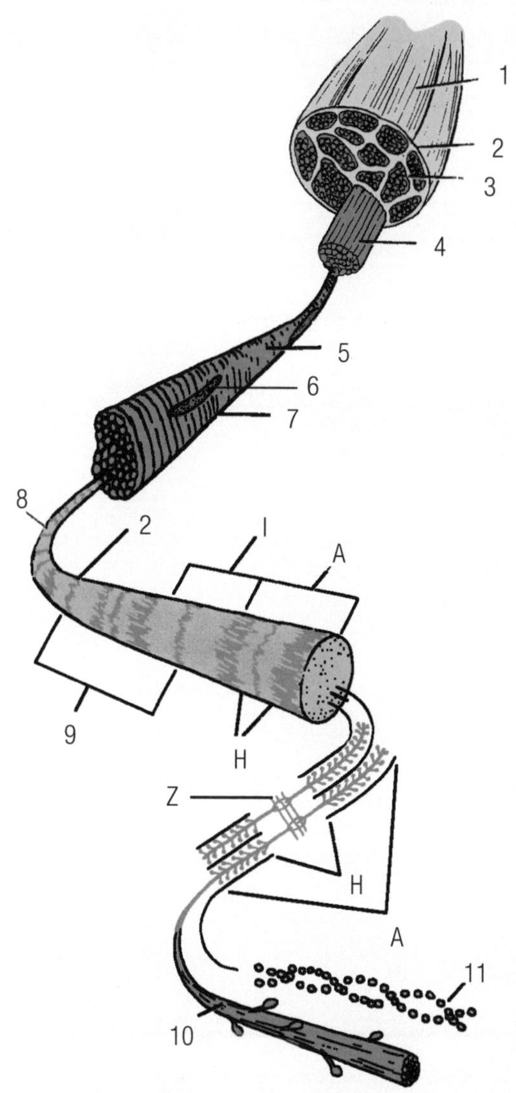
1
2
3
4
5
6
7
8
2
I
A
9
H
Z
H
A
11
10

Neuromuscular Junction –
Nerve end attaching to Skeletal muscle
longitudinal

1 axon – *sheathed*
2 mylein sheath – *multiple lipid layers*
3 Schwann cell
4 axonlemma – *axon membrane*
5 pre-synaptic vesicles
6 axon – *unsheathed / naked*
7 presynaptic membrane
8 junctional folds *(in sarcolemma)*
9 synaptic cleft *(~20nm)*
10 mitochondria
11 sarcolemma
12 myofilaments *in muscle fibre*

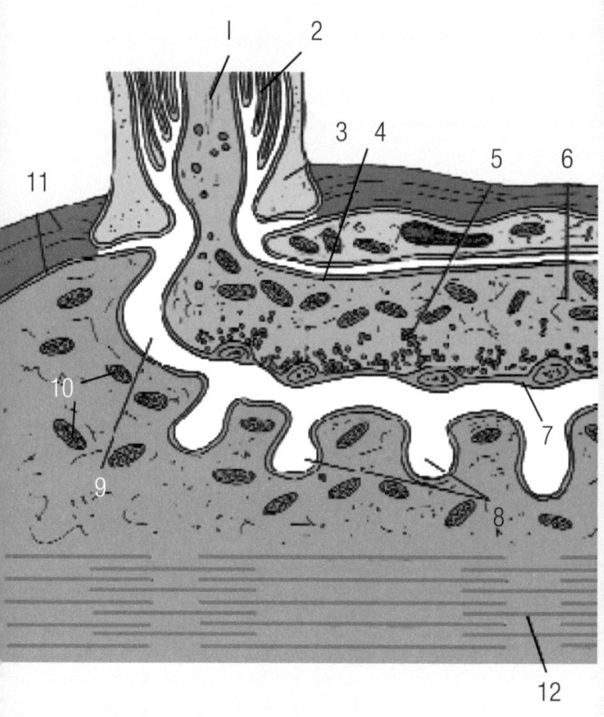
1
2
3
4
5
6
11
10
9
7
8
12

Neuro-Muscular Spindle –

feedback loop to stop overextension in Skeletal muscle

Neuro-Tendinous Spindle –

feedback loop to stop overextension in the tendon

1 capsule of spindle
2 myelinated motor fibres
3 myelinated sensory fibres
4 unmyelinated motor fibres
5 annualospiral fibre endings
6 bag of nuclei *in intrafusal muscle*
7 motor end plates
8 muscle fibres i = intrafusal e = extrafusal
9 skeletal muscle nuclei
10 tendon fibres i = intrafusal e = extrafusal
11 naked axons
12 nuclei in tendon

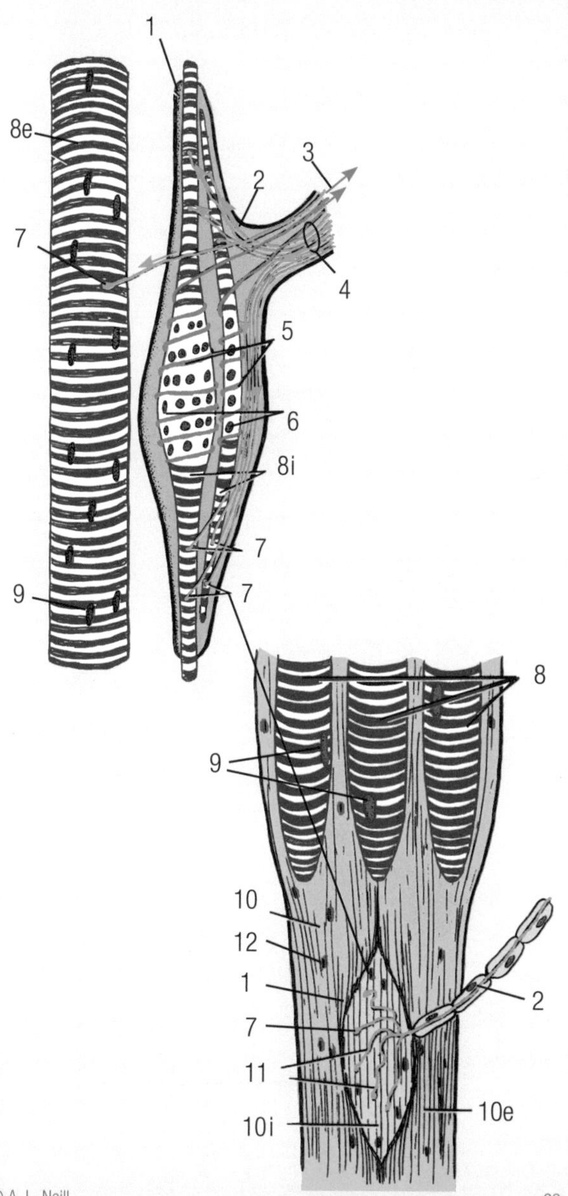
1
8e
3
2
7
4
5
6
8i
7
9
7
8
9
10
12
1
2
7
11
10e
10i

Anatomical Planes and Relations

This is the anatomical position.

A= Anterior Aspect from the front Posterior Aspect from the back used interchangeably with ventral and dorsal respectively

B= Lateral Aspect from either side

C= Transverse / Horizontal plane

D= Midsagittal plane = Median plane; trunk moving away from this plane = lateral flexion or lateral movement moving into this plane medial movement; limbs moving away from this direction = abduction; limbs moving closer to this plane = adduction

E= Coronal plane

F= Median

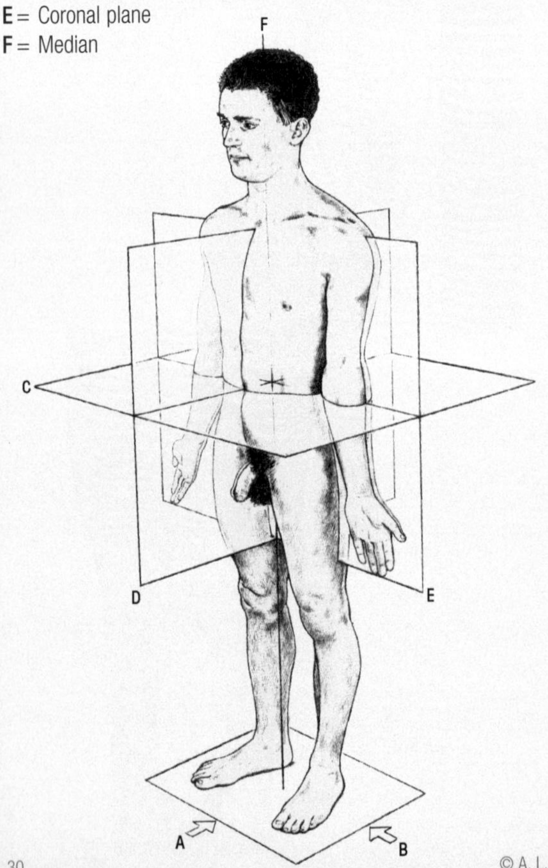

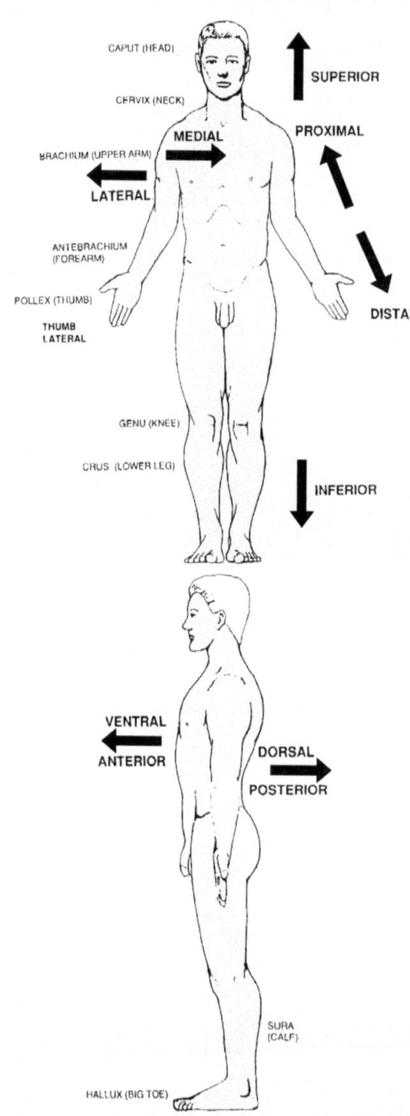
CAPUT (HEAD)
SUPERIOR
CERVIX (NECK)
MEDIAL
PROXIMAL
BRACHIUM (UPPER ARM)
LATERAL
ANTEBRACHIUM
(FOREARM)
POLLEX (THUMB)
THUMB
LATERAL
DISTAL
GENU (KNEE)
CRUS (LOWER LEG)
INFERIOR
VENTRAL
ANTERIOR
DORSAL
POSTERIOR
SURA
(CALF)
HALLUX (BIG TOE)

Anatomical Movements

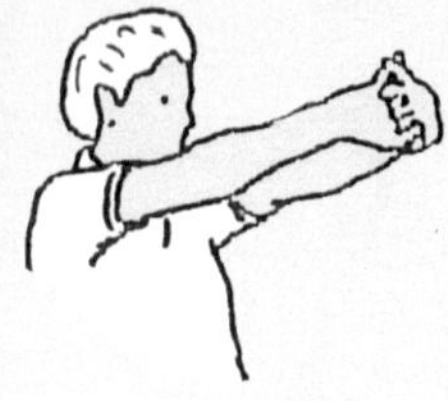

arm extension in sagittal plane / shoulder movement

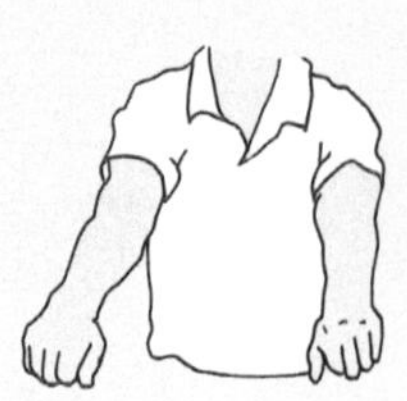

arm abduction -away from median plane / adduction-towards the median plane -shoulder movement

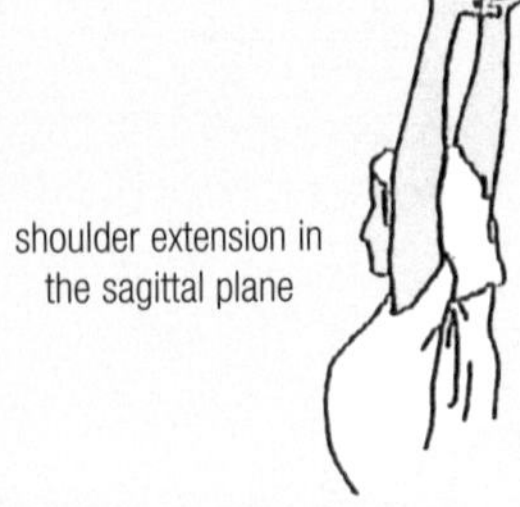

shoulder extension in the sagittal plane

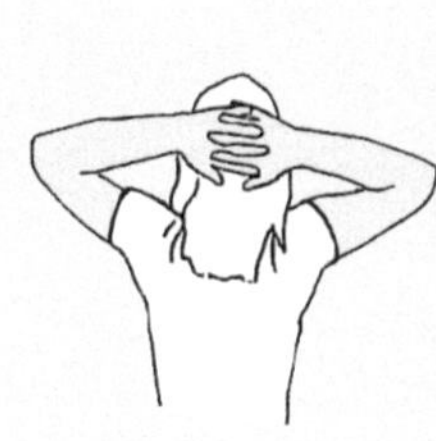

shoulder abduction in the coronal plane (with elbow flexion)

shoulder elevation
- reverse movement shoulder depression
shoulder movement

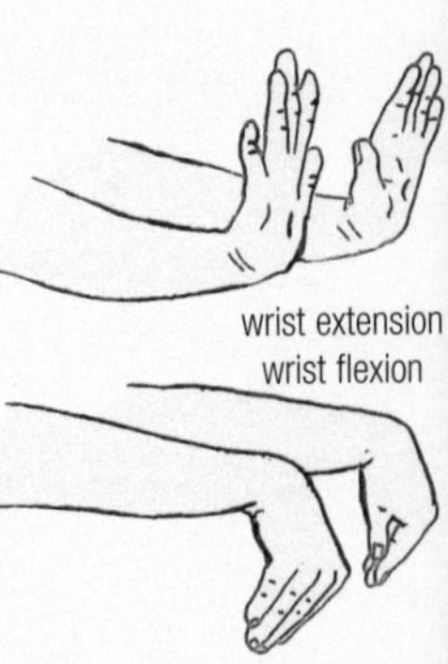

wrist extension
wrist flexion

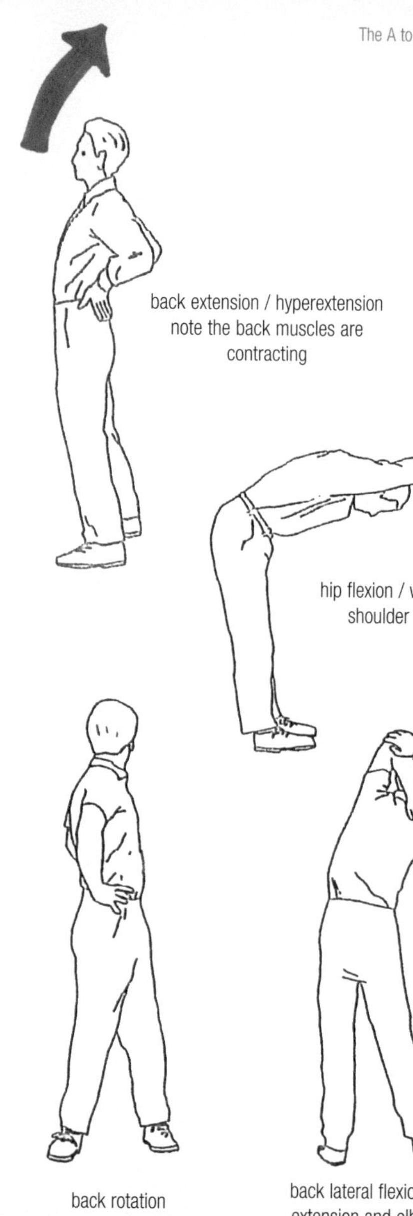

back extension / hyperextension
note the back muscles are
contracting

hip flexion / with back and
shoulder extension

back rotation

back lateral flexion shoulder
extension and elbow flexion

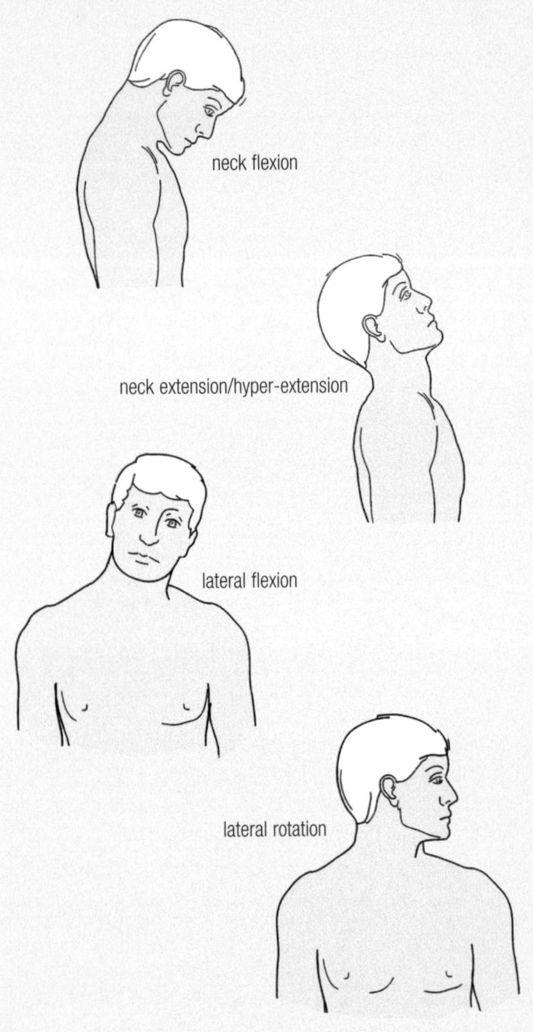

note: extension of the neck is in the normal anatomical position

arm/shoulder movements in the coronal plane commencing from adduction abduction to extension

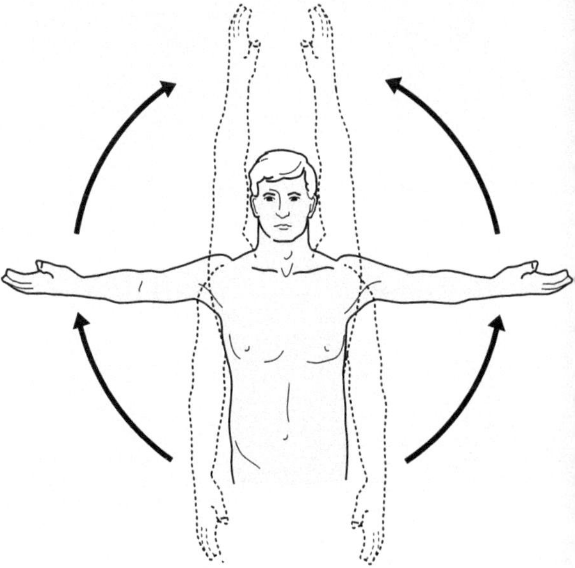

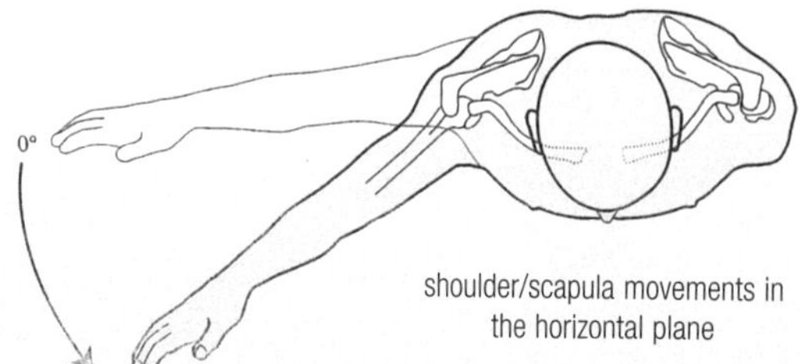

shoulder/scapula movements in the horizontal plane

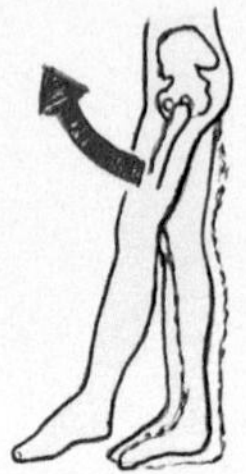
Hip flexion

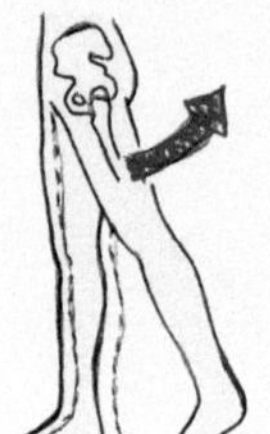
Hip extension

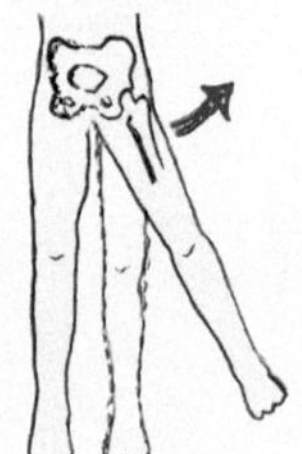
Hip abduction

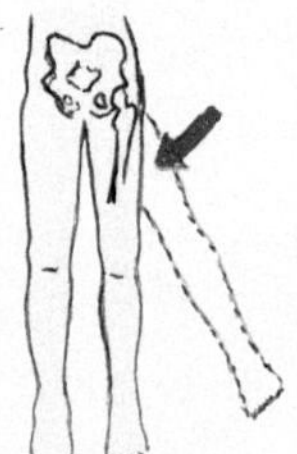
Hip adduction

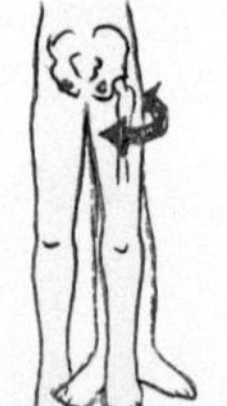
Hip lateral and medial rotation

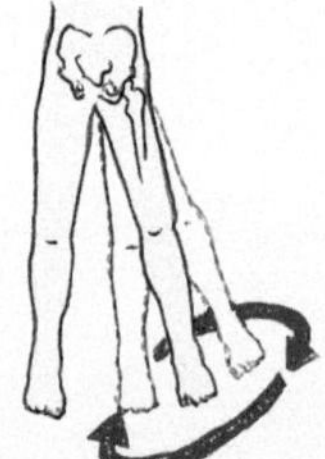
Hip circumduction

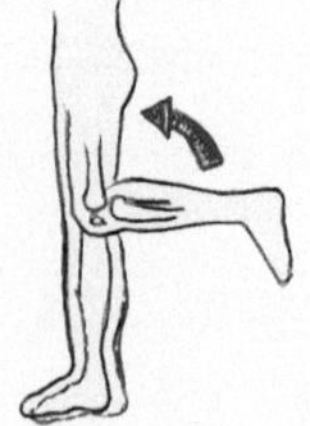
Knee flexion

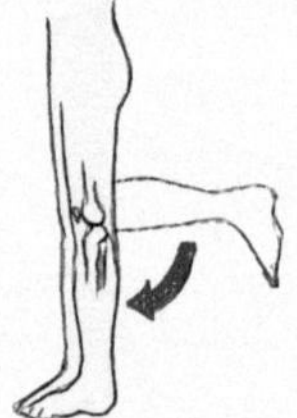
Knee extension

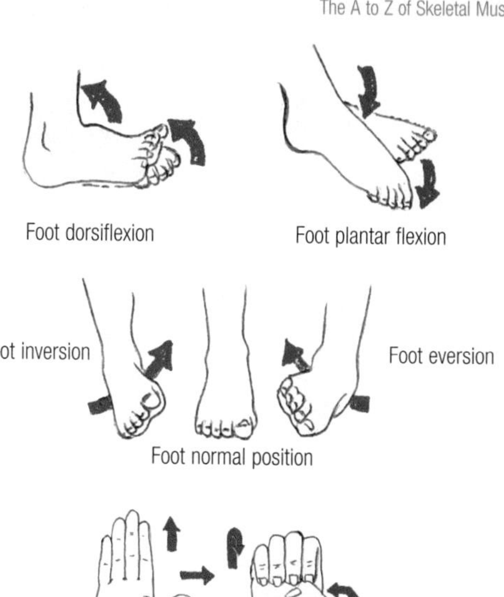

Foot dorsiflexion

Foot plantar flexion

Foot inversion

Foot normal position

Foot eversion

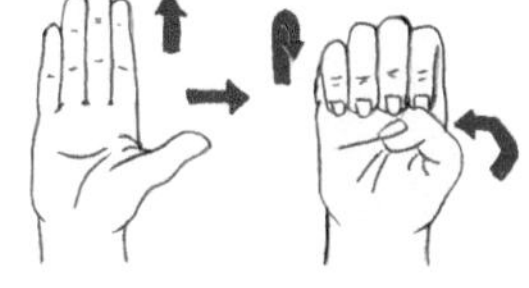

Fingers extension

Fingers flexion

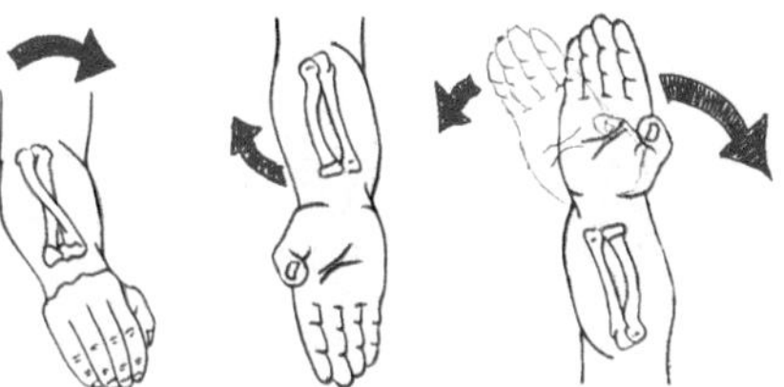

Forearm pronation

Forearm supination

Hand deviation radial/ laterally ulna/medially

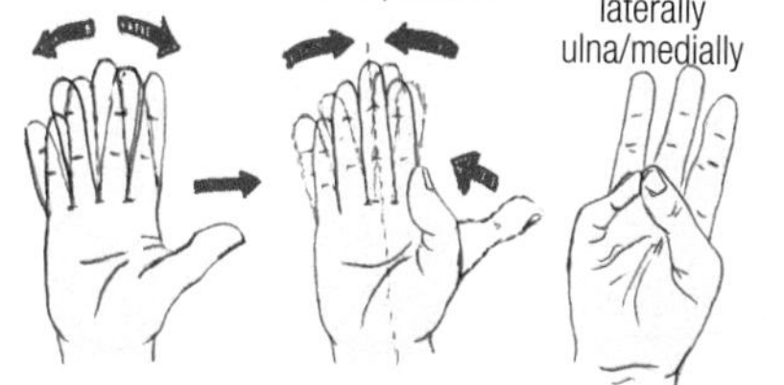

Fingers abduction

Fingers adduction

Thumb opposition

Foot Movements

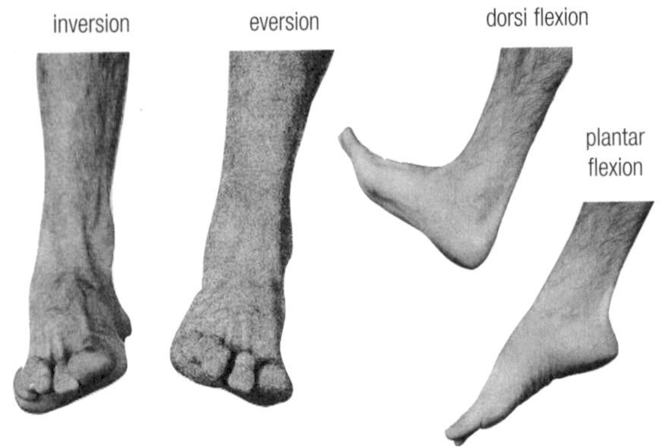

Hand Movements & Grips

The hand & wrist may be involved in a huge range of different grips & fine specialized movements calling upon a combination of muscles to allow for the precision of the actions.

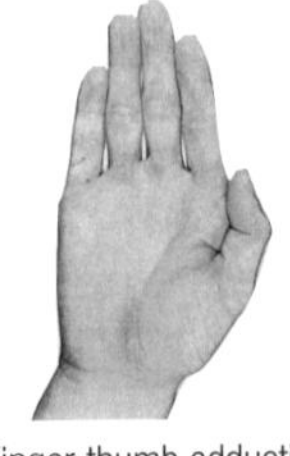

Finger thumb adduction
Dorsal Interossei

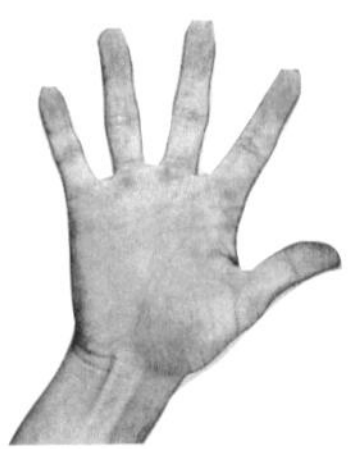

Finger thumb abduction
Palmar Interossei

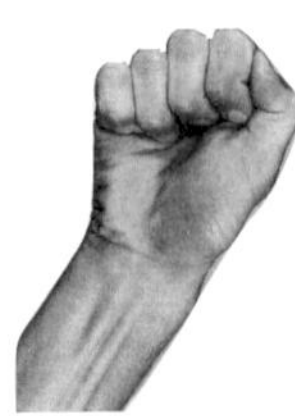

Finger thumb flexion
FDP, FPL

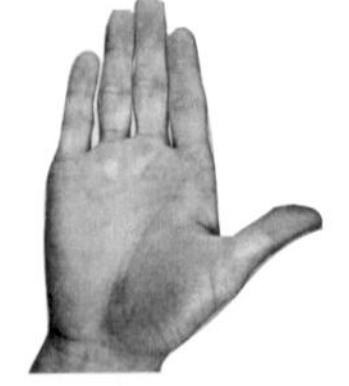

Finger thumb extension ant. dorso-lat *(anat snuff box) ED, EP*

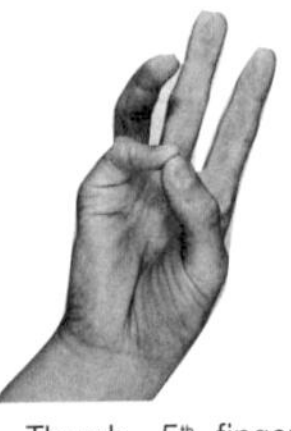

Thumb - 5th finger opposition *TE, HE, OP*

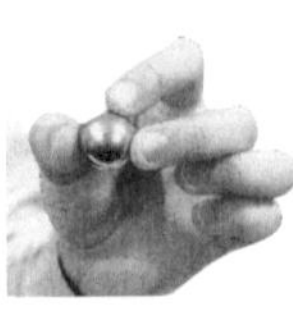

Opposition/flexion
Carpal curve for precision grip

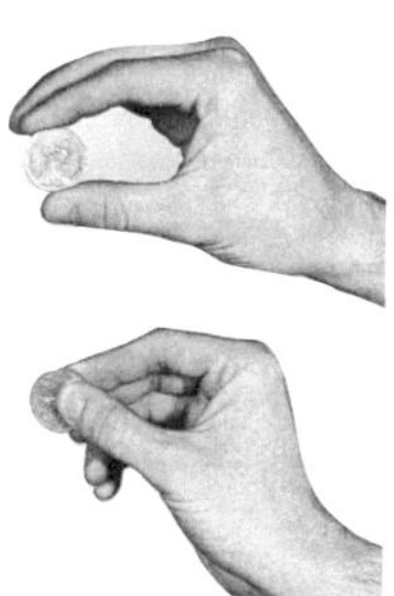

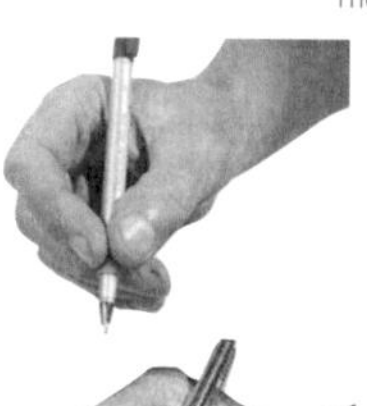

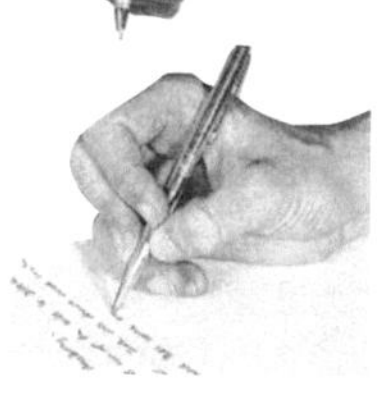

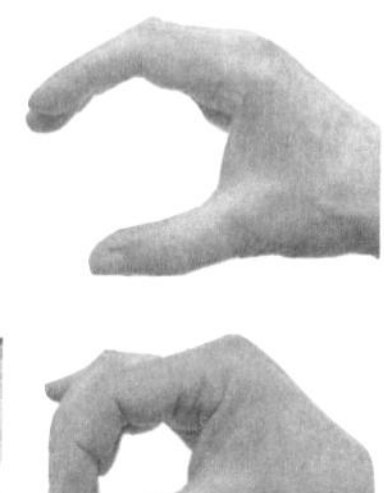

Thumb index – precision grip *TE, HE, OP*

Thumb fingers - ± intrinsic hand muscles writing grip - precision *interossei*

Open grip, Pinch lat.

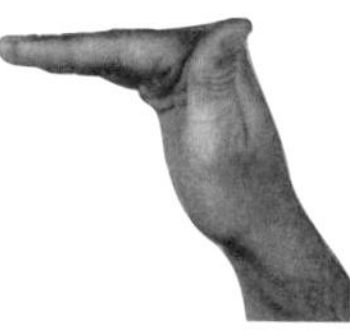

Finger extension - hand flexion *Lumbricles*

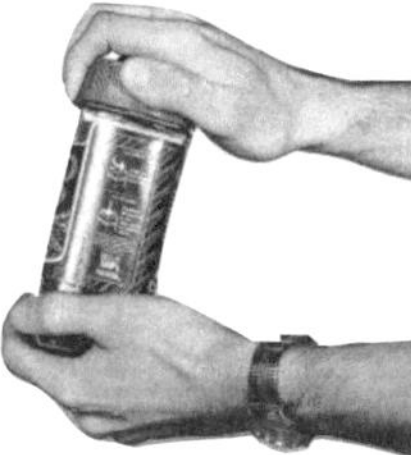

Hands coordinate in 2 handed procedures – unscrewing

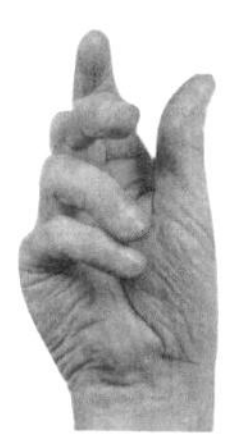

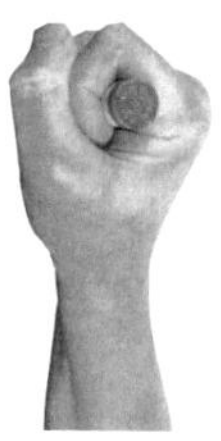

Power grips making use of friction - finger tips, PB HE+ TE for additional grip also boney curves - carpal curve shape of the phalanges

Practical holds demonstrating power grip variations

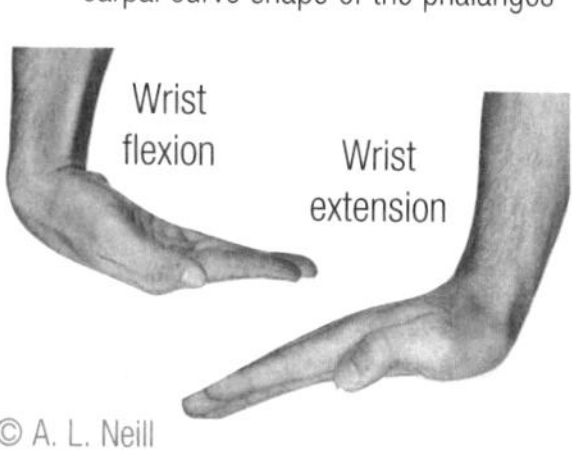

Wrist flexion

Wrist extension

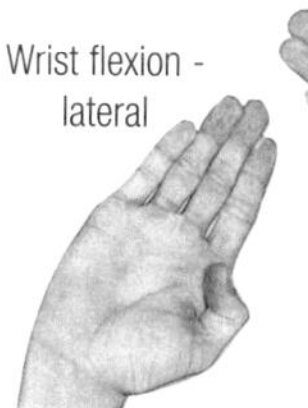

Wrist flexion - lateral

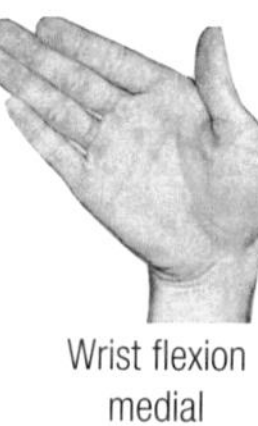

Wrist flexion medial

Classification, Naming & Examination of Muscles

There are 3 types of muscle tissue and this book discusses only one of them SKELETAL MUSCLE. The other 2 are smooth muscle (for the gut and other areas of involuntary movement) and cardiac muscle (for the heart).

SKELETAL muscle is defined as muscle which is "striated" or striped, indicating and ordered cell structure, of myosin and actin filaments, and is generally under voluntary control, which has an action on the skeleton or bones in the body.
In its relaxed form the muscle is at its maximum length and this is generally how the tissue is found. Stimulation generally causes contraction and a shortening and thickening of the tissue. As it is attached to a minimum of 2 points, the Origin (O) and the insertion (I) - although these may be arbitrarily named - this "contraction" brings these 2 points closer together. To reverse this, another muscle must be attached to 2 different points which when they move together cause a reversal of the position of the 2 or more affected bones, hence for each muscle there is an antagonist (opposing muscle) and in many situations a synergist (a muscle which enhances the original movement).

There are a few exceptions to this, for example SPHINCTERS are circular groups of muscle fibres which upon contraction close the circle they have formed and may not be attached to bones at all. Their function is to prevent leakage or passage of material from one area to another.
Many of the MUSCLES OF FACIAL EXPRESSION are inserted into the deep fascia of the skin and hence change the soft tissues of the face but do not affect the bones underneath. We as humans have a great deal of these muscles, and they may be shifted or injured in many cosmetic procedures because of this structure.

Muscle are shaped to allow their contraction to occur in the most efficient manner, for example sheets of muscles cover expanses of tissue to contain them, as in the OBLIQUES to contain and move bulky abdominal contents, or DIAPHRAGMS to separate as well as move large anatomical regions around, while TERES muscles are small, cordlike, focused groups of fibres for very specific movements.
Generally the smaller the muscles the deeper they are placed so larger and more powerful muscles ones can cover them, for example the GLUTEAL and ADDUCTOR group of muscles in the leg and buttocks. Smaller muscles generally have more specific actions, are more resilient but are weaker, they contract and relax repeatedly for example, to maintain posture or balance, as in the ROTATORES. Larger, longer muscles by definition cannot be as precise but have larger ranges of motion and more power and are placed more superficially - closer to the surface, as in ERECTOR SPINAE.

Fibrous tissue inserts give the muscle more strength but less ability to move, as in RECTUS ABDOMINUS versus TRAPEZIUS, but it is these large surface/ superficial muscles whose shape can be changed and defined by gross movement exercises.

Muscles are named using many different criteria singly or in combination: for example they may be named according to their action –Supinator, Pronator and size – Adductor Magnus, Adductor Longus, Adductor Brevis; their shape and location- Biceps Brachii, Triceps Brachii, Quadratus Lumborum, Interossei, Intercostals; the direction of their muscle fibres and anatomical layer - Obliquus Externus Abdominus, Obliquus Internus Abdominus and there does not seem to be a consistent pattern in this naming - only that from the name it is often possible to determine their site, action &/or shape and this helps when memorizing these muscles.

Between each muscle group is a fascial layer to transport in the BVs and the Nerves but there is considerable variation in individuals so that in some cases some anatomists have named the same muscle in several ways. The commonest has been used here but the alternatives listed if it is thought there may be confusion this for example ROTATORES has been listed as a single muscle group but may in some books be divided into 2 ROTATORES LONGUS and BREVIS, similarly with PSOAS which can be PSOAS MAJOR and MINOR, but not with PECTORALIS MAJOR and MINOR, 2 distinct muscles. Wherever this occurs it is mentioned in the text, particularly if there is a functional difference in the 2 muscles.

M0	no active contraction
M1	palpable contraction – but no movement
M2	weak contraction – not strong enough to counter gravity
M3	contraction can overcome gravity
M4	contraction – enables function but is not full strength
M5	full strength

S0	absence of all sensory modalities
S1	deep pain sensation
S2	recovery of protective sensation, generalized – heat, pain, touch
S3	recovery of localized sensation / and recognition of objects
S4	normal sensation

Myotomes

Each muscle is supplied by a particular NR or segment of the SC and the muscles supplied by the same NR belong to the same MYOTOME. These are briefly grouped as follows.

- C1,2 neck and upper VC muscles
- C3-5 diaphragm
- C5 shoulder and upper arm
- C6 wrist extension
- C7 extension of the elbow
- C8 finger movement
- T1 finger abduction
- T1-12 chest and abdominal muscles
- L1,2 hip flexion
- L3 knee extension
- L4 foot dorsiflexion
- L5 toe movement
- S1 plantar flexion of the foot
- S2-5 organs of the pelvis and perineum including bladder and bowel and genitals

These muscles are listed in detail in the following table.

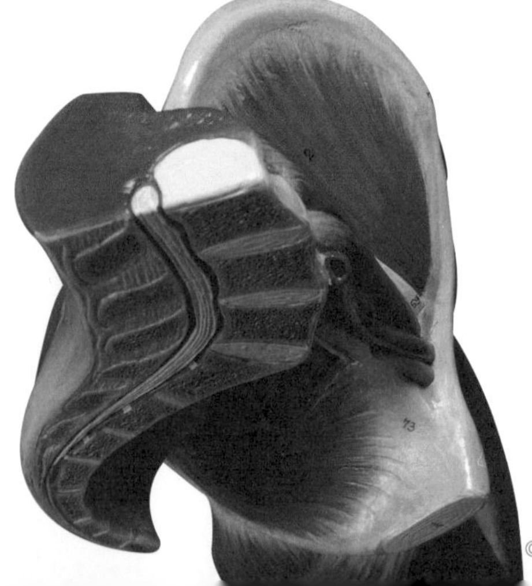

Muscle innervation at the SC level

SC level	Muscle	Location
C1	Longus Capitus	Neck
	Olquuis Capitus Superior	Neck - head
	Rectus Capitus Anterior	Neck - head
	Rectus Capitus Major	Neck - head
	Rectus Capitus Minor	Neck - head
	Semispinalis Capitus	Neck - head
	Trapezius	Back
C2	Longus Capitus	Neck
	Longus Colli	Neck - head
	Rectus Capitus Anterior	Neck - head
	Semispinalis Capitus	Neck - head
	Sternocleidomastoid	Neck - head
	Trapezius	Back
C3	Levator Scapulae	Neck - shoulder
	Longus Capitus	Neck
	Longus Colli	Neck - head
	Semispinalis Capitus	Neck - head
	Rhomboideus Major	Back - shoulder
	Rhomboideus Minor	Back - shoulder
	Sternocleidomastoid	Neck - head
	Trapezius	Back
C4	Iliocostalis Cervicis	Neck - chest
	Levator Scapulae	Neck - shoulder
	Longus Capitus	Neck
	Longus Colli	Neck - head
	Rhomboideus Major	Back - shoulder
	Rhomboideus Minor	Back - shoulder
	Sternocleidomastoid	Neck - head
	Trapezius	Back
C5	Brachialis	Arm
	Brachioradialis	Arm
	Biceps Brachii	Arm
	Deltoid	Shoulder - arm
	Iliocostalis Cervicis	Neck - chest
	Infraspinatus	Neck - shoulder
	Levator Scapulae	Neck - shoulder
	Longus Capitus	Neck
	Longus Colli	Neck - head
	Pectoralis Major	Chest - arm
	Rhomboideus Major	Back - shoulder
	Rhomboideus Minor	Back - shoulder
	Scalenus Ant. Medial &Post.	Neck
	Semispinalis Capitus	Neck - head
	Semispinalis Cervicus	Neck
	Serratus Anterior	Chest
	Sternocleidomastoid	Neck - head
	Subscapularis	Shoulder
	Supraspinatus	Shoulder

	Teres Major	Arm - back
	Teres Minor	Arm - back
	Trapezius	Back
C6	Abductor Pollicis Longus	Hand - thumb
	Brachialis	Arm
	Brachioradialis	Arm
	Biceps Brachii	Arm
	Coracobrachialis	Arm - elbow
	Deltoid	Shoulder - arm
	Extensor Carpi Radialis Brevis	Forearm - wrist
	Extensor Carpi Radialis Longus	Forearm - wrist
	Extensor Carpi Ulnaris	forearm - wrist
	Extensor Digitorum	Hand - fingers
	Extensor Digiti Minimi	Hand - little finger
	Extensor Indicis	Hand - index finger
	Extensor Pollicis Brevis	Hand - thumb
	Extensor Pollicis Longus	Hand - thumb
	Flexor Carpi Radialis	Wrist
	Iliocostalis Cervicis	Neck - chest
	Infraspinatus	Neck - shoulder
	Latissimus Dorsi	Back - arm
	Longus Colli	Neck - head
	Pectoralis Major	Chest - arm
	Pronator Teres	Forearm - wrist
	Scalenus Anterior	Neck - head
	Scalenus Medial	Neck - head
	Scalenus Posterior	Neck - head
	Semispinalis Capitus	Neck - head
	Semispinalis Cervicus	Neck
	Serratus Anterior	Chest - arm
	Subscapularis	Scapula - shoulder
	Supinator	Forearm - wrist
	Supraspinatus	Neck -shoulder
	Teres Major	Arm - chest
	Trapezius	Back
C7	Abductor Pollicis Longus	Hand - thumb
	Anconeus	Elbow-Arm-Forearm
	Brachialis	Arm
	Brachioradialis	Arm
	Coracobrachialis	Arm - elbow
	Extensor Carpi Radialis Brevis	Forearm - wrist
	Extensor Carpi Radialis Longus	Forearm - wrist
	Extensor Carpi Ulnaris	forearm - wrist
	Extensor Digitorum	Hand - fingers
	Extensor Digiti Minimi	Hand - little finger
	Extensor Indicis	Hand - index finger
	Extensor Pollicis Brevis	Hand - thumb
	Extensor Pollicis Longus	Hand - thumb
	Flexor Carpi Radialis	Wrist
	Flexor Digitorum	Hand - fingers
	Iliocostalis Cervicis	Neck - chest
	Infraspinatus	Neck - shoulder
	Latissimus Dorsi	Back - arm
	Longus Colli	Head - neck

	Pectoralis Major	Chest - arm
	Pronator Teres	Forearm - wrist
	Scalenus Anterior	Neck - head
	Semispinalis Cervicus	Neck
	Serratus Anterior	Chest - arm
	Subscapularis	Scapula-shoulder
	Supinator	Forearm - wrist
	Supraspinatus	Neck - shoulder
	Teres Major	Arm - chest
	Trapezius	Back
	Triceps Brachii	Arm - elbow
C8	Abductor Digiti Minimi	Hand - little finger
	Abductor Pollicus Brevis	Hand - thumb
	Abductor pollicus Longus	Hand - thumb
	Adductor Pollicus	Hand - thumb
	Anconeus	Elbow
	Dorsal Interossei	Hand - fingers
	Extensor Carpi Ulnaris	Wrist
	Extensor Digitorum	Hand - fingers
	Extensor Digiti Minimi	Hand - little finger
	Extensor Indicis	Hand - index finger
	Extensor Pollicis Longus	Hand - thumb
	Flexor Carpi Ulnaris	Wrist
	Flexor Pollicus Brevis	Hand - thumb
	Flexor Pollicus Longus	Hand - thumb
	Iliocostalis Cervicus +Thoracis	
	Lumbricals	Hand - fingers
	Opponens Pollicis	Hand - thumb
	Palmar Interossei	Hand - fingers
	Pectoralis Major	Thorax - chest
	Pronator Quadratus	Hand
T1	Abductor Digiti Minimi	Hand - little finger
	Abductor Pollicus Brevis	Hand - thumb
	Adductor Pollicus	Hand - thumb
	Dorsal Interossei	Hand - fingers
	Flexor Carpi Ulnaris	Wrist
	Flexor Ddigitorum Profundus	Hand - fingers
	Flexor Digitorum Superficialis	Hand - fingers
	Flexor Pollicus Brevis	Hand - thumb
	Flexor Pollicus Longus	Hand - thumb
	Lumbricals	Hand - fingers
	Opponens Digiti minimi	Hand - little finger
	Opponens Pollicis	Hand - thumb
	Palmar Interossei	Hand - fingers
	Pectoralis Major	Thorax - chest
	Pronator Quadratus	Hand
L2	Adductor Brevis	Hip - thigh
	Adductor Longus	Hip - thigh
	Adductor Magnus	Hip - thigh
	Gracilis	Hip - thigh
	Iliacus	Hip - thigh
	Pectineus	Hip
	Rectus Femoris	Hip - thigh - knee

	Sartorius	Hip - thigh - knee
	Vastus Intermedius	
	Vastus Lateralis	Hip - thigh - knee
	Vastus Medialis	Hip - thigh - knee
L3	Adductor Brevis	Hip - thigh
	Adductor Longus	Hip - thigh
	Adductor Magnus	Hip - thigh
	Gracilis	Hip - thigh
	Iliacus	Hip - thigh
	Pectineus	Hip
	Rectus Femoris	Hip - thigh - knee
	Sartorius	Hip - thigh - knee
	Vastus Intermedius	
	Vastus Lateralis	Hip - thigh - knee
	Vastus Medialis	Hip - thigh - knee
L4	Adductor Brevis	Hip - thigh
	Adductor Longus	Hip - thigh
	Adductor Magnus	Hip - thigh
	Extensor digitorum Brevis	Foot - toes
	Extensor Digitorum Longus	Foot - toes
	Extensor Hallucis Longus	Foot - big toe
	Gemellus Inferior	Hip
	Gluteus Medius	Hip
	Gluteus Minimus	Hip
	Gracilis	Hip - thigh
	Iliacus	Hip - thigh
	Obturator Externus	Hip - pelvis
	Pectineus	Hip
	Peroneus Brevis	Leg - ankle
	Peroneus Longus	Leg - ankle
	Popliteal	Knee
	Quadratus Femoris	Hip - thigh - knee
	Rectus Femoris	Hip - thigh - knee
	Tibialis Anterior	Leg - ankle
	Vastus Intermedius	Hip - thigh - knee
	Vastus Lateralis	Hip - thigh - knee
	Vastus Medialis	Hip - thigh - knee
L5	Biceps Femoris	Hip - thigh
	Extensor Digitorum Brevis	Foot - toes
	Extensor Digitorum Longus	Foot -toes
	Extensor Hallucis Longus	Foot - big toe
	Flexor Digitorum Brevis	Foot - toes
	Flexor Digitorum Longus	Foot - toes
	Flexor Hallucis Longus	Foot - big toe
	Gemellus Inferior	Hip
	Gemellus Superior	Hip
	Gluteus Maximus	Hip
	Gluteus Medius	Hip
	Gluteus Minimus	Hip
	Lumbrical (first)	Toe
	Obturator Externus	Hip - pelvis
	Oburator Internus	Hip - pelvis
	Pectineus	Hip

	Peroneus Brevis	Leg - ankle
	Peroneus Longus	Leg - ankle
	Popliteal	Knee
	Quadratus Femoris	Hip - thigh - knee
	Semimembranous	Hip - thigh - knee
	Semitendinous	Hip - thigh - knee
	Tensor fascia Lata	Hip - leg
	Tibialis Anterior	Leg - ankle
	Tibialis Posterior	Leg - ankle
S1	Biceps Femoris	Hip - thigh
S1	Extensor Digitorum Longus	Foot - toes
	Extensor Hallucis Longus	Foot - big toe
	Flexor Digitorum Brevis	Foot - toes
	Flexor Digitorum Longus	Foot - toes
	Flexor Hallucis Longus	Foot - big toe
	Gastrocnemius	Knee - leg
	Gemellus Inferior	Hip
	Gemellus Superior	Hip
	Gluteus Maximus	Hip
	Gluteus Medius	Hip
	Gluteus Minimus	Hip
	Lumbrical (first)	Toe
	Obturator Externus	Hip - pelvis
	Oburator Internus	Hip - pelvis
	Pectineus	Hip
	Peroneus Brevis	Leg - ankle
	Peroneus Longus	Leg - ankle
	Piriformis	Hip
	Quadratus Femoris	Hip - thigh - knee
	Semimembranous	Hip - thigh - knee
	Semitendinous	Hip - thigh - knee
	Tensor fascia Lata	Hip - leg
	Tibialis Anterior	Leg - ankle
	Tibialis Posterior	Leg - ankle
S2	Biceps Femoris	Hip - thigh
	Flexor Hallucis Longus	Foot - big toe
	Gastrocnemius	Knee - leg
	Gemellus Superior	Hip
	Gluteus Maximus	Hip
	Lumbricals (2-4)	Toes
	Oburator Internus	Hip - pelvis
	Piriformis	Hip
	Semimembranous	Hip - thigh - knee
	Semitendinous	Hip - thigh - knee
	Soleus	Foot - toes
S3	Lumbricals (2-4)	Toes

Segmental Motor Diagram

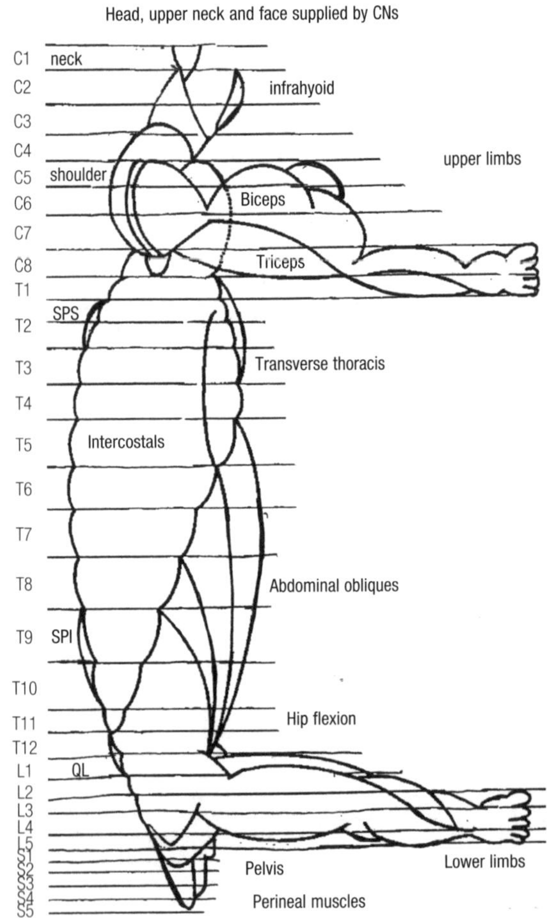

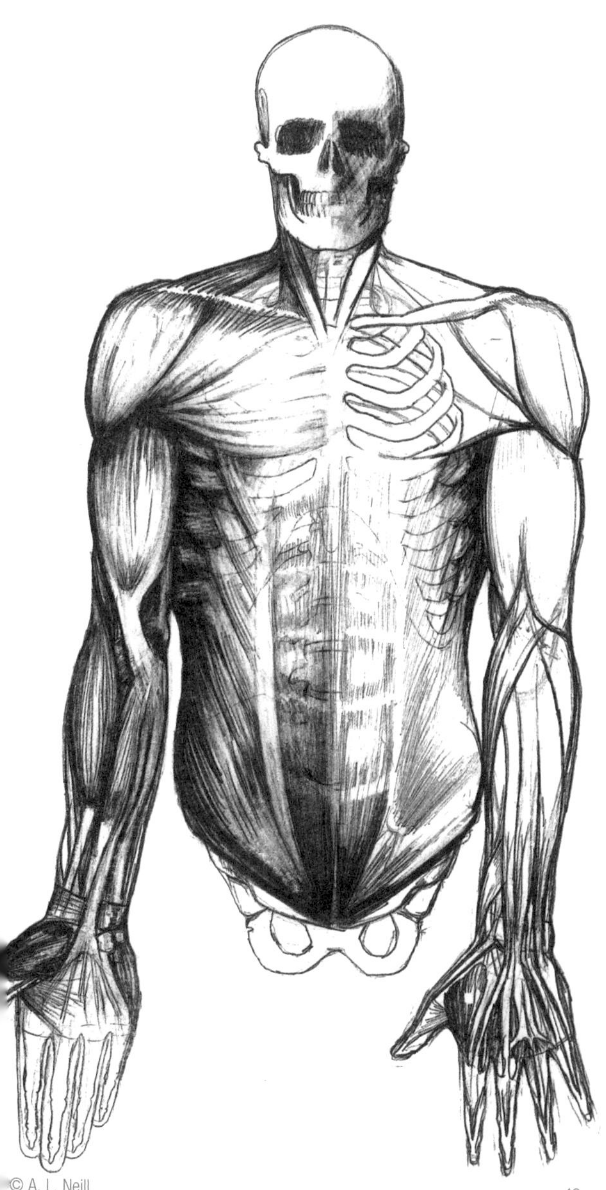

Summaries of Skeletal Muscle Groups

Muscles of the arm
Muscles of the arm and shoulder

Deltoid
Rotator Cuff muscles Subscapularis, Supraspinatus, Infraspinatus, Teres Major & Minor

NS from the **BP – C5-7**
BS from the axillary artery & branches

External Rotators = Lateral Rotators

Infraspinatus Teres Minor

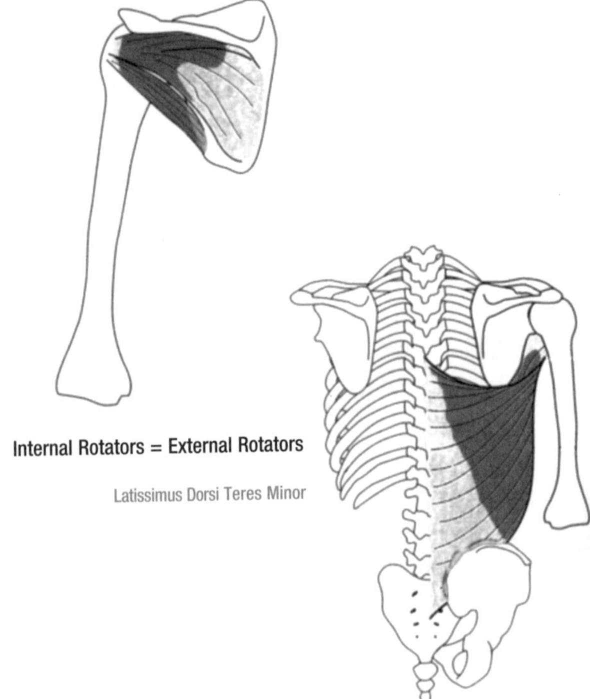

Internal Rotators = External Rotators

Latissimus Dorsi Teres Minor

Muscles connecting the arm with the VC

Levator Scapulae
Rhomboids Major & Minor
Trapezius
Latissimus Dorsi

NS segmental (C2-T12)
BS from dorsal branches of the aorta

Muscles connecting the arm with the chest wall

Pectoralis Major & Minor
Serratus Anterior
Subclavius

segmental **NS** and **BS** from the axillary and long thoracic

Muscles in the anterior compartment of the arm - flexors

Biceps Brachii
Coracobrachialis
Brachialis

NS musculocutaneous (C5-6)
BS brachial

Muscles in the posterior compartment - extensors

Triceps Brachii

NS radial (C7-8)
BS profunda brachii and branches

Muscles of the forearm

anterior

superficial
Pronator Teres
Palmaris Longus
Flexor Carpi Radialis
Flexor Carpi Ulnaris

intermediate
Flexor Digitorum Superficialis

deep
Flexor Pollicis Longus
Flexor Digitorum Profundus
Pronator Quadratus

NS median and ulnar Ns - **BS** radial branches

posterior

superficial
Extensor Digitorum
Extensor Digiti Minimi
Extensor Carpi Ulnaris
Anconeus

deep
Supinator
Abductor Pollicis Longus
Extensor Pollicis Longus & Brevis
Extensor Indicis

NS radial (C7-C8)
BS radial and interosseous branches

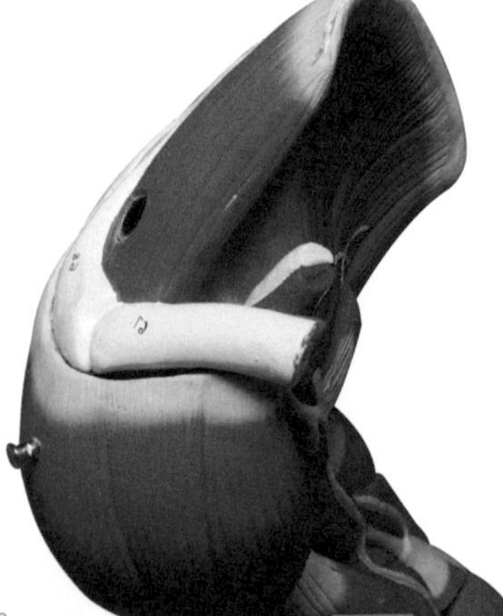

** For details of these layers and to see the muscles in s go to* ***The A to Z of Surfa Anatomy***

Intrinsic muscles of the hand

THENAR EMINENCE (Side of the thumb)
Muscles: Abductor Pollicus Brevis
Flexor Pollicus Brevis
Opponens Pollicus

NS: median, C8
BS: median, medial of Superfical and Deep Palmer anastomoses

HYPOTHENAR EMINENCE (Side of the little finger)
Muscles: Abductor Digiti Minimi
Flexor Digiti Minimi
Oppons Digiti Minimi

NS: ulnar, T1
BS: ulnar, lateral of Superfical and Deep Palmer anastomoses

OTHER
Muscles: Adductor Pollicus
Lumbricals (4)
Interossei (7-8)
Palmar and Dorsal

BS: ulnar and radial, palmar anastomoses and digital branches

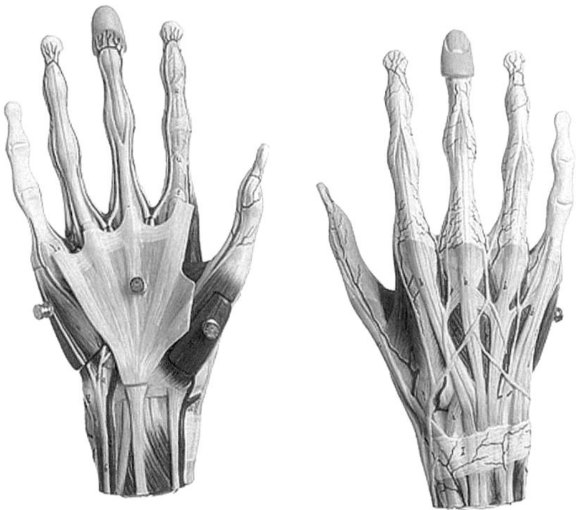

* *For details of these muscles in situ go to* ***The A to Z of Surface Anatomy***

Muscles of the Hip and Buttocks (Gluteal region)

Gluteus Maximus, Medius, Minimus

Lateral – External Rotators

1 Obturator Externus
2 Obturator Internus
3 Gemellus Inferior
4 Quadratus Femoris
5 Gemellus Superior
6 Piriformis

Medial – Internal Rotators

7 Gluteus Minimus
8 Tensor Fascia Lata (part of the ITB)

NS local L4-S2

BS superior gluteal

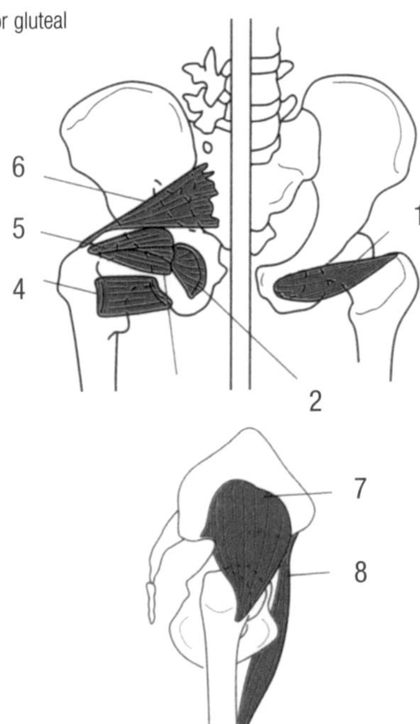

Muscles of the gluteal region

Muscles:

Gluteus Maximus
Medius and Minimus
Piriformis
Superior and Inferior Gemellus
Obturator Internus
Quadratus Femoris

NS: local, L4-S2
BS: superior gluteal

Muscles and muscle layers of the chest and abdomen

superficial
Pectoralis Major & Minor
Serratus Anterior & Posterior
Rectus Abdominus
middle
External & Internal Intercostals
External & Internal Obliques
deep
Innermost Intercostals
Levator Costi Longus & Brevis
Tranversus Thoracics
Transverses Abdominus
Quadratus Lumborum

NS segmental (C3-L2)
BS from C3-L2

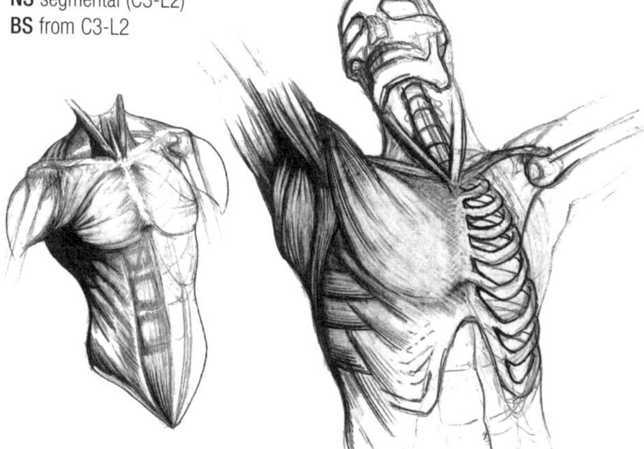

Muscles of the Hip and Thigh

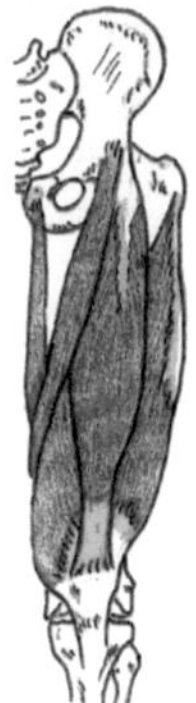

anterior compartment muscles - hip flexors / knee extensors

Sartorius
Iliopsoas
Pectineus
Quadriceps Femoris = Vastus Intermedius +
V. Lateralis V. Medialis + Rectoris Femoris (deep)

NS femoral N (L2-5)
BS femoral

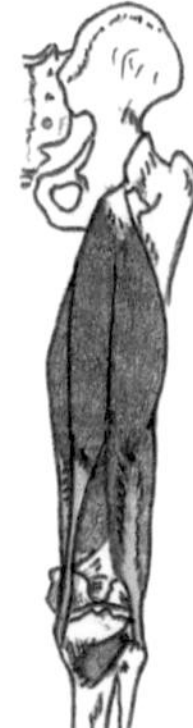

posterior compartment muscles - hip extensors /knee flexors

Hamstrings = Semimembranous +
Semitendinous + Biceps Femoris
Adductor Magnus

NS sciatic N (L2-S2)
BS profunda femoris

medial compartment muscles - hip adductors

Gracilis
Adductor Magnus, Longus, Brevis
Obturator Externus
Pectineus

NS obturator N (L2-4)
BS obturator, profunda femoris

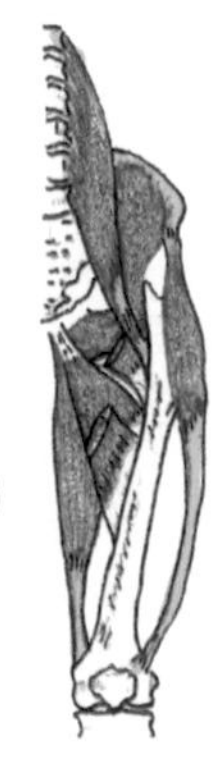

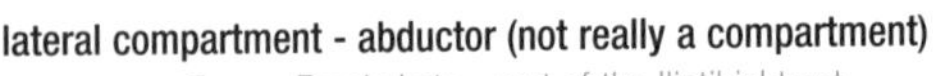

lateral compartment - abductor (not really a compartment)

Tensor Fascia Lata - part of the Iliotibial tract

NS superior gluteal (L4-S1)
BS superior gluteal, lateral femoral circumflex

Muscles of the leg

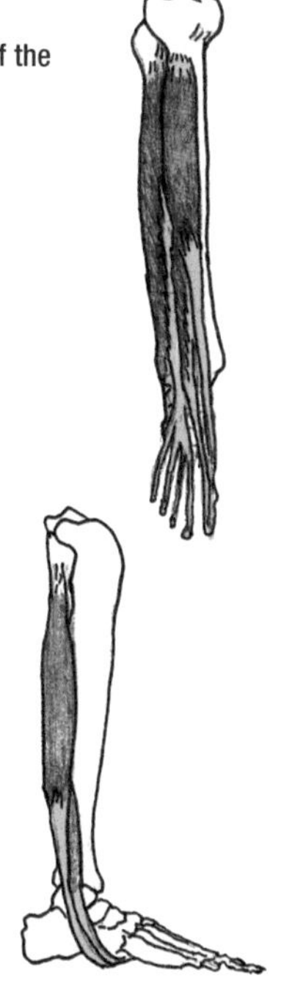

anterior compartment muscles - dorsi-flexors of the ankle, extensors of the toes

Extensor Digitorum Longus
Extensor Hallicus Longus
Peroneus Tertius
Tibialis Anterior

NS deep peroneal N (L5-S1)
BS anterior tibial

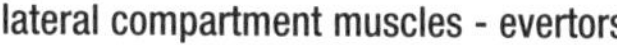

lateral compartment muscles - evertors

Peroneus Brevis. Longus

NS superficial peroneal N (S1-2)
BS peroneal

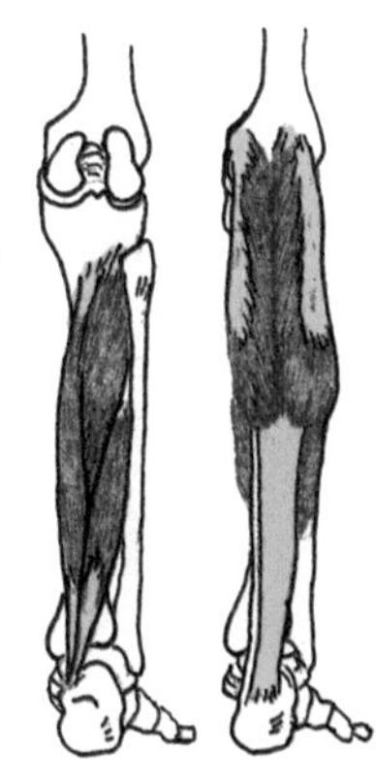

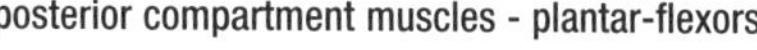

posterior compartment muscles - plantar-flexors

superficial Gastrocnemius, Plantaris, Soleus
deep Extensor Digitorum Longus
Flexor Hallicus Longus, Popliteus
Tibialis Posterior

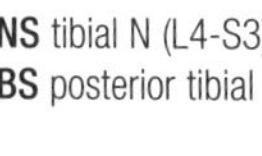

NS tibial N (L4-S3)
BS posterior tibial

Intrinsic muscles of the sole of the foot*

Dorsal surface of the foot - dorsi-flexors

Extensor Digitorum Brevis

Extensor Hallicus Brevis and Dorsal Interossei (intrinsic muscles of the foot) and the tendons of the Longus Extensors cross over this surface (not shown).

NS deep peroneal N (S1-2)
BS dorsalis pedis

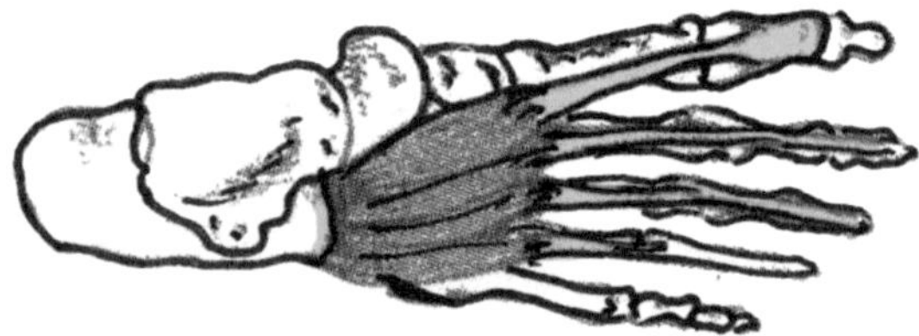

Plantar surface
superficial layer - closest to the surface of the sole of the foot

Abductor Hallicus

Flexor Digitorum Brevis

Abductor Digiti Minimi

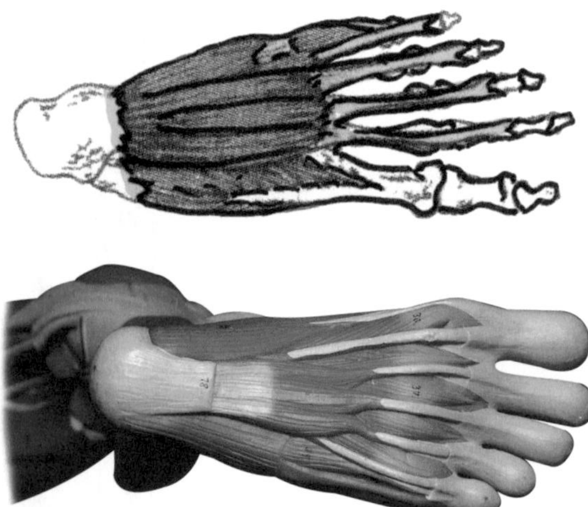

Details of the foot muscle layers including plantar aponeurosis are found in* ***The A to Z of Surface Anatomy*

second layer

Quadratus Plantae
Lumbricals and tendons of the Flexors of the toes and big toe

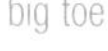

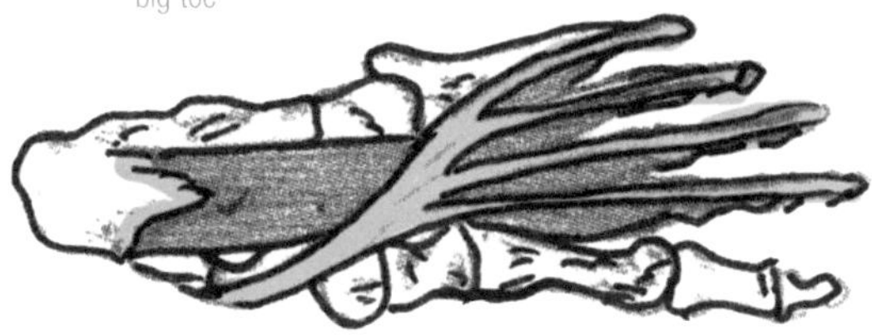

third layer

Flexor Hallicus Brevis
Adductor Hallicus
Flexor Digiti Minimi

fourth and deepest layer of the sole - closet to the bones

Interossei
Tendons of Peroneus Longus and Tibialis Posterior

NS lateral plantar (S1-3)
BS lateral plantar

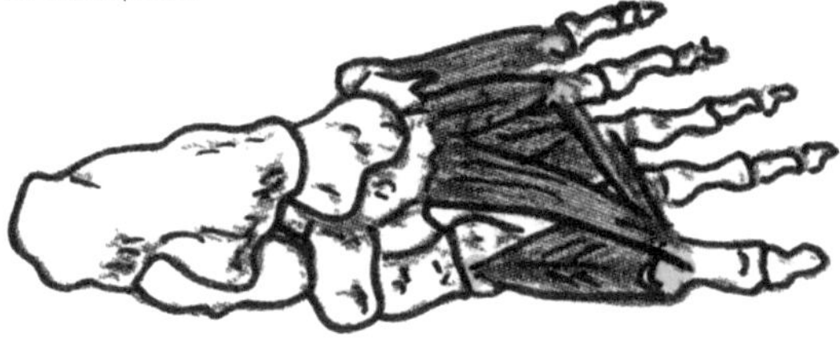

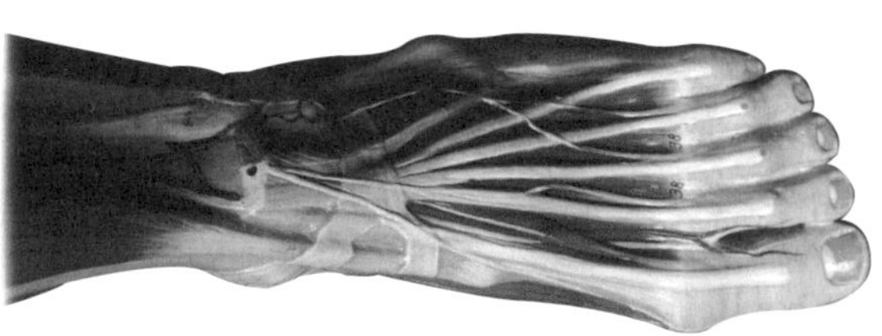

Muscles of the Lower Limb

Transverse, Lower leg = leg, Upper leg = thigh

This schema shows a transverse section through the upper and lower leg, and the relationship with the compartments which are much more defined in the LL than in the UL. Compression will result in muscle death

1 Tibia
2 Great Saphenous vein & N
3 Extensor Digitorum longus (e) + Flexor Digitorum Longus (f)
4 neurovascular bundles – travelling in fascial planes
5 subcut. fat supf to the deep fascia investing the muscles
6 Soleus M
7 peroneal art & vein
8 Extensor Hallicus longus (e) Flexor Hallicus Longus (f)
9 deep fascia extensions to demarcate the compartments of the LL i = interosseous membrane (leg only)
ii - iii post. compartment leg - medial compartment thigh
iii - iv lat. compartment leg - post compartment thigh
iv – ii ant. compartment leg & thigh #
10 Peroneus brevis (b), Peroneus longus (L)
11 Fibula
12 supf peroneal N
13 Sartorius M
14 Tibialis
a = anterior
p = posterior
15 obturator N
16 Gracilis M
17 semimembranous M
18 Semitendinous M
19 Biceps Femoris M
20 Adductors / b = brevis / L = longus / m = magnus
21 sciatic N
22 Gluteus maximus M
23 Femur
24 Vasti muscles
i = intermedius /
m = medialis /
l = lateralis
25 Rectus femoris

**Note compression of the ant. compartment will result in compression of this nv*

 # note small lat compartment of thigh with Tensor Fascia Lata not shown

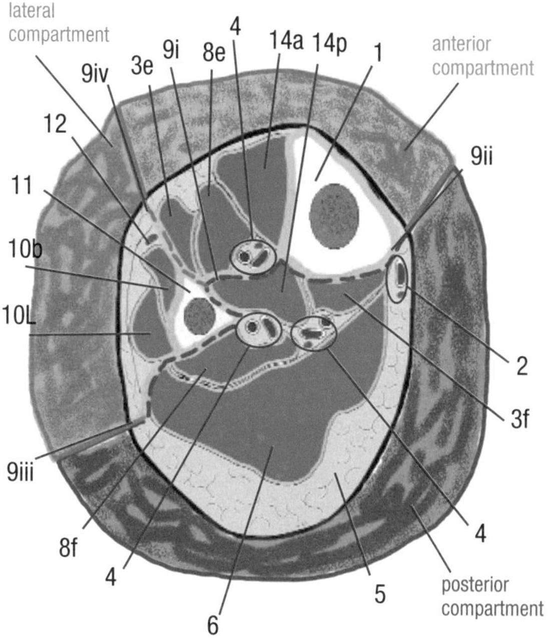

lateral compartment
4
14a
14p
1
anterior compartment
9i
8e
3e
9iv
12
9ii
11
10b
10L
2
3f
9iii
8f
4
4
5
posterior compartment
6

anterior compartment
24
25
4
13
24
4
9ii
medial compartment
24
16
23
15
20b
20m
9iv
9iii
17
posterior compartment
22
18
21
19

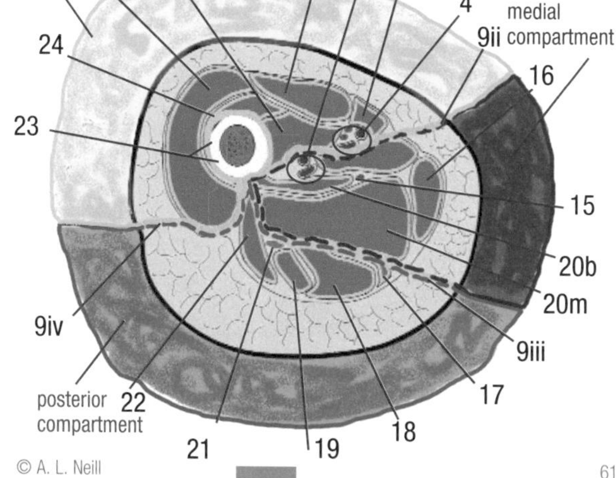

Muscles of the Neck

NECK – has 2 major groups of muscles

1 those concerned with the neck movement
i.e. movement of the cervical spine & head

2 those concerned with the anterior neck structures i.e. the larynx & pharynx.

Group 1

deep posterior - suboccipital muscles – extensors / hyperextensors/rotators and stabilizers

Rectus Capitus Posterior – Major and Minor
Obliquuis Capitus muscles
Cervical & Cephalic / Capitus regions of the muscles of the VC (5, 6)

NS segmental - dorsal rami of the related SNs
BS dorsal branches of the carotids

deep anterior - prevertebral flexors, rotators and stabilizers

Rectus Capitus ant. & lat. (1, 10)
Longus Colli supporting mainly the cervical vertebrae (8) and
Longus Capitus (9) supporting mainly the head

NS segmental - ventral rami of related SNs
BS branches of carotids and other local vessels
These muscles are covered by the prevertebral fascia of the neck.

anterior - flexors, rotators

Scalenii muscles -anterior, medial and posterior (7)

NS segmental anterior branches of the ventral rami
BS superficial cervical

These muscles are covered by the prevertebral fascia of the neck.

1 Rectus capitus lateralis
2 Splenius capitus
3 Digastricus – post belly
4 Levator scapulae
5 Longissimus cervicus
6 Iliocostalis cervicus
7 Scalenes a = ant , m = middle p = post
8 Longus colli
9 Longus capitus
10 Rectus capitus anterior
11 Mastoid and styloid processes
12 Ribs 1 & 2
13 ALL
14 Sphenoid
15 EAM
16 Occiput

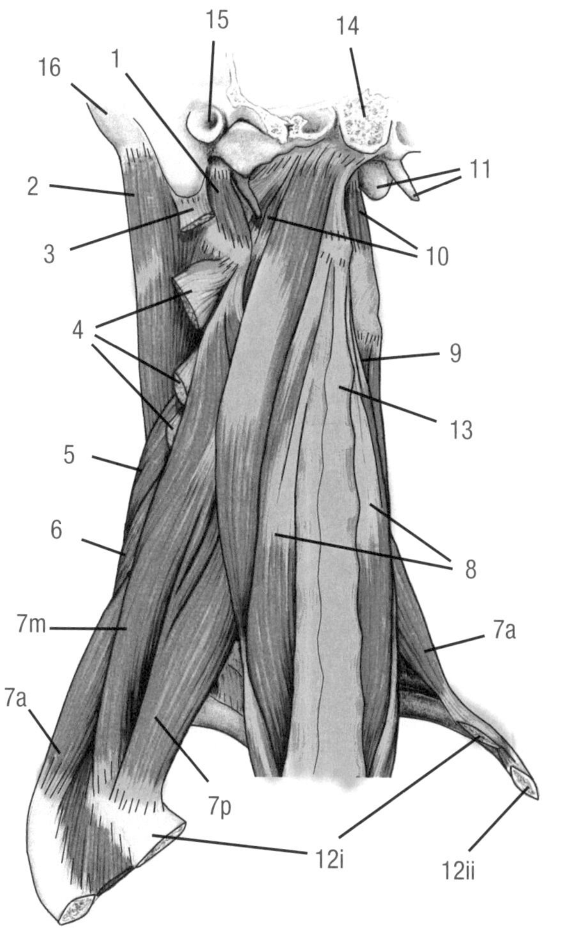
15
14
16
1
11
2
3
10
4
9
13
5
6
8
7m
7a
7a
7p
12i
12ii

Anterior of the root of the neck relations with the ANS, Brachial plexus and Great Vessels

1 vertebral artery (L)
2 TP of CI (Atlas) (L)
3 superior cervical ganglion (L)
4 Levator Scapulae M
5 Scalenus Medius M
6 phrenic N (N roots C3,4,5)
7 Scalenus Anterior M
8 upper trunk of the BP (L)
9 thyrocervical trunk and deep cervical branch
10 inferior cervical ganglion
11 Thoracic duct
12 subclavian vessels (L)
13 Sternothyroid (L) M
14 Trachea
15 hyoid muscles (R) = Sterno- hyoid thyroid
16 common carotid artery
17 CN X = Vagus N
18 Omohyoid M
19 BP = brachial plexus
20 Oesophagus
21 TP of C6 (anterior tubercle)
22 middle cervical ganglion (R)
23 sympathetic trunk
24 Longus Colli M

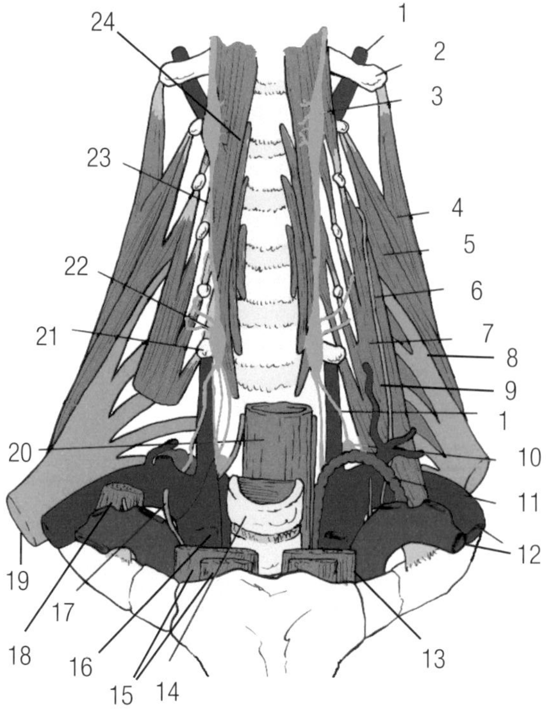
24
1
2
3
23
4
5
22
6
21
7
8
9
1
20
10
11
12
19
17
18
16
15
14
13

Transverse section C7 relations with the cervical fascial layers, VC and anterior neck structures

Transverse section C7

1 skin, subcutaneous tissue, superficial fascia
2 SP of C7
3 deep fascia & investing layers
4 Trapezius M
5 Splenius M
6 Spinalis M
7 loose CT / with LNs + vessels / autonomic ganglion / BVs
8 Transverse foramen + Vertebral artery
9 Platysma M
10 Sternocleidomastoid M
11 External Jugular vein
12 anterior neck muscles / strap muscles
13 Anterior Jugular vein
14 Trachea + cartilagenous ring and surrounding fascia
15 Thyroid
16 Oesophagus
17 Carotid sheath and contents = common carotid art. + internal jugular vein + Vagus N
18 Pretracheal fascia
19 deep muscles of the neck and back = Rotatores, Multifidus, Intertransversarii
20 SC - Nervous tissue + coverings

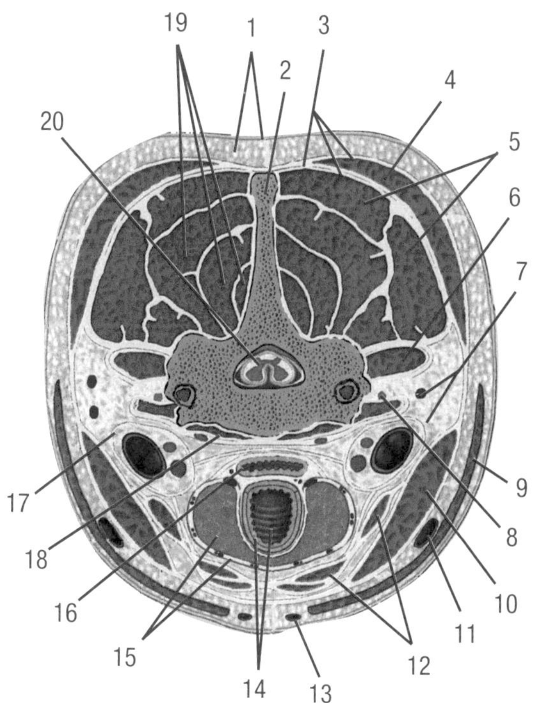
19
1
3
2
4
20
5
6
7
17
9
18
8
16
10
11
15
12
14
13

BACK - has 2 major groups of muscles

1 those which are intrinsic to the VC basically segmental muscles concerned with movements and stability of the VC particularly the deepest layers - connected with the movement of the neck etc.
2 those which use the VC as an immoveable post and move structures around the back extrinsic concerned with the anterior neck structures.

EXTRINSIC

muscles which move the shoulder and arm
Trapezius, Latissimus Dorsi, Rhomboids
Levator Scapulae
muscles which move the rib cage
Serratus Posterior inferior and superior

NS segmental - ventral rami of related SNs
BS branches of carotids and other local vessels

INTRINSIC

most superficial
Erector Spinae - ES divided into a number of muscle groups with regional distinctions
medial →lateral
Spinalis Iliocostalis Longissimus
Iliocostalis - Lumborum, Thoracis, Cervicus
Longissimus - Thoracis, Cervicus, Capitus
Spinalis - Thoracis, Cervicus, Capitus

O & I listed individually in the text
as a group
O along the VC, Sacrum and Ribs
I into the VC and Ribs
A *listed individually*
A as a group the ES extends and rotates the VC
NS - segmental spinal roots generally the dorsal rami but may alos have innervation from the dorsal branches of the ventral rami branches (C1-L5) - cervical and capitus regions act upon the neck
BS - segmental dorsal branches of the descending aorta, lumbar and sacral arteries
T - to stand up from touching toes w/o help
- from upright position bend to one side and the other w/o help

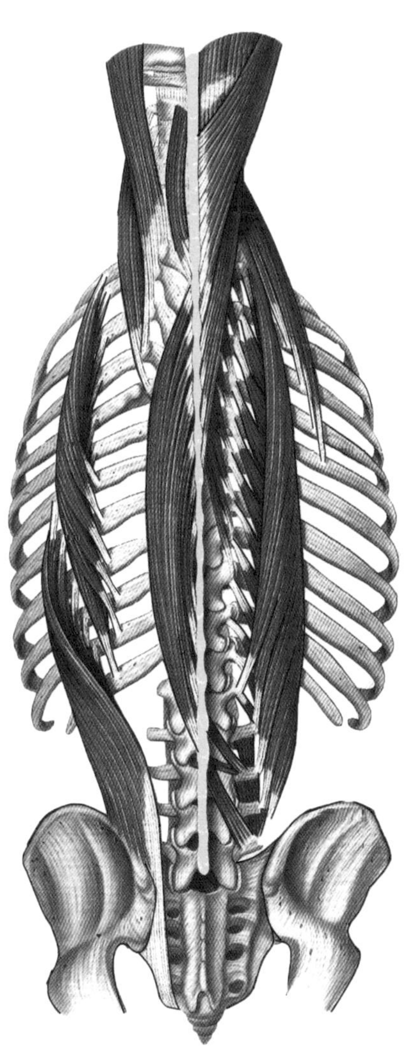

The summary below is brief and only an overview of these muscles for completeness of this muscle book. They are discussed in individual detail in *The A to Z of Surface Anatomy.*

Muscles of the Perineum

(only female anatomy shown)

Anterior - urogenital triangle bordered by the pubic arch and ischeal tuberosities and overlaid by the structures of the Vulva.
Bulbospongiosus surrounding the urethra and vagina combined and compressing their orifices during coitus
Ischiocavernosus encasing glandular tissue which contacts in coitus to expel the contents
Sphincter Urethrae = Urethral Sphincter
sphincter hence circular muscle inserting all around
natural position - constricted rather than relaxed
Transverse Perineal - Profundus between the perineal fascae, Superficialis
these muscles overlie each other with the
perineal diaphragm in b/n
Superficialis - inferior to Profundus hence closer to the skin

NS pudendal (S2-4)
BS pudendal

Posterior - anal triangle bordered by the ischeal tuberosities and the coccyx
Coccygeus from the isheal spine tom the coccyx
Levator Ani = Pubococcygeus + Iliococcygeus
Sphincter Ani = External Anal Sphincter Ischiococcygeus
sphincter hence circular muscle inserting all around
natural position - constricted rather than relaxed

A muscles of this region act to support the pelvic contents and the perineum and are intimately related so that damage to any of this basin of tissue will have profound effects on the functional capacities of the others.

NS pudendal and Ns from SP (S2-4)
BS internal iliacs

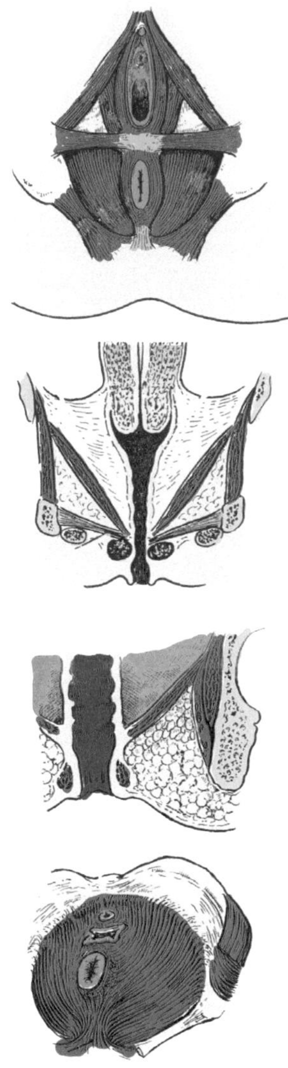

Muscles of the Eye

Note all 6 of these muscles act "in concert" in eye movement and depend upon the fixation and focus of the eye, included is the muscle which moves the eyelid to follow the eye gaze, hence 6+1.

Extrinsic

Muscles responsible for movement of the upper eyelid

1 Levator Palpebrae Superioris
NS oculomotor N (CN III)
BS supraorbital, branches of ophthalmic N (from CN V_1)

Muscles responsible for movement of the eyeball

2 Recti muscles - Inferior/Superior, Medial/Lateral.
These muscles are straight and are responsible for one movement up/down, in/out

3 Oblique muscles - Inferior, Superior
These muscles are attached via a trochlea 3t or pulley and movements therefore vary on eye position and are diagonal up and out/ down and in

All are attached to the scleral surface, the Recti via the optic canal on the common annular tendon, (5) & the Obliques via bones in the optic cavity (6)

NS oculomotor N (CNIII) - except Lateral Rectus - abducent N (CN VI) (CNVI) and Superior Oblique - trochlea N (CN IV)
BS ophthalmic and branches of internal carotid

Note the CN responsible for vision is the Optic N CN II (8) which exits from the back of the pupil through the optic canal

Intrinsic

These muscles are responsible for moving structures within the eyeball and are not shown but affect the lens (9) and iris (7).

NS Oculomotor N (CN III) parasympathetic outflow
BS ophthalmic and branches of internal carotid

10 Ciliaris
11 Dilator Pupillae
12 Sphincter Pupillae

The cornea (13) is a modified form of the CT which forms the sclera and the ciliary body (14) attaches long strands of connecting fibres (15) which affect the curvature of the lens.

* *For more details see* ***The A to Z of the Head and Neck.***

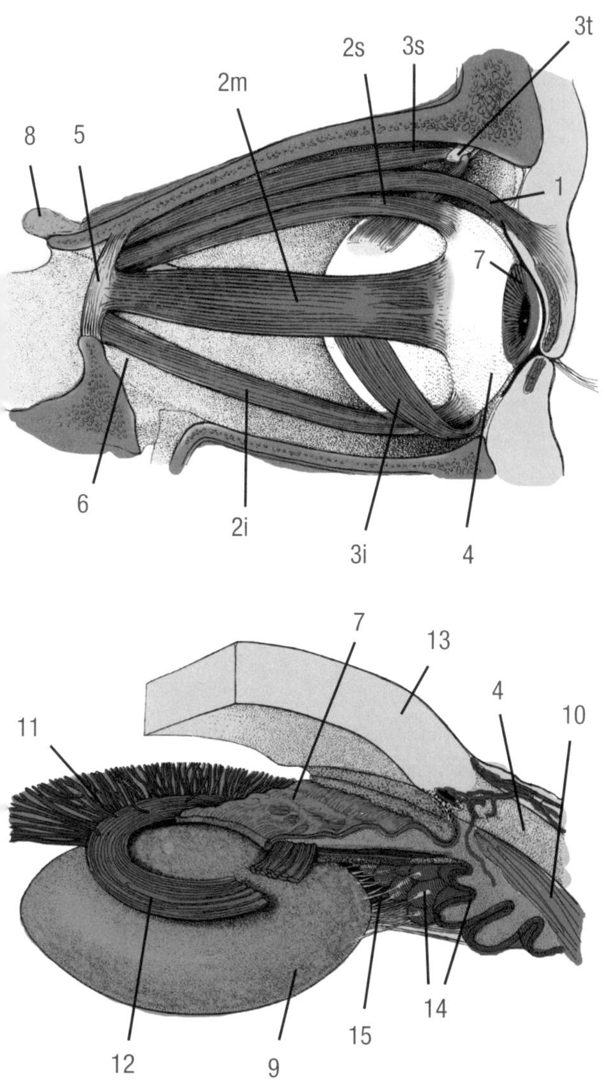
3t
2s
3s
2m
8
5
1
7
6
2i
3i
4
7
13
4
10
11
12
9
15
14

Muscles of the Eye

in situ

removal of superficial tissue / coronal section / enucleation with muscle bed intact

1 Levator palpebrae superioris
2 4 x recti muscles (superior, inferior, lateral, medial)
3 2 x oblique muscles (superior, inferior)
4 Trochlear N (CN IV)
5 Ciliary ganglion (CN III)
6 Abducens N (CN VI)
7 Oculomotor N + branches (CN III)
8 Trochlea
9 Superior orbital notch
10 Superior orbital fissure
11 Optic N (CN II)
12 Lacrimal gland

see orbital cavity for bony orbit P48

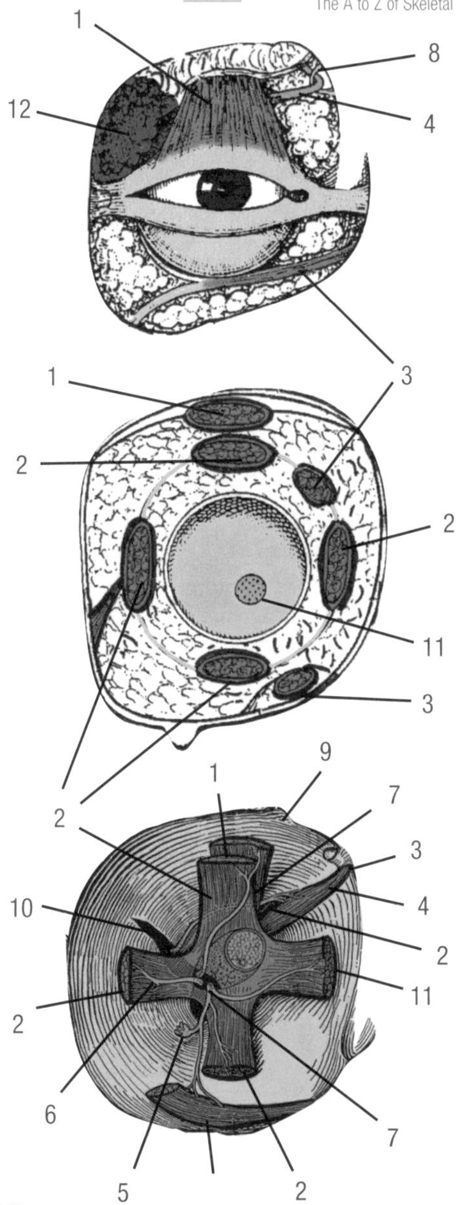
1
8
12
4
3
1
2
3
2
11
3
2
2
9
1
7
2
3
4
10
2
2
11
2
6
7
5
2

Face – muscles of expression and lip and cheek movement

Anterior – major muscles of the face

1 Frontalis muscle belly

2 Temporalis

3 muscles of the nose
c = Compressor naris
d = Dilator naris
s = Depressor septi nasi

4 4L Levator anguli oris
4D Depressor anguli oris

5 Masseter

6 Buccinator

7 Risorius

8 Orbicularis oris

9 Depressor labii inferioris

10 Mentalis

11 Platysma 2 bellies – on both the lower face &neck

12 split in the Platysma may widen with age leading to softening and heaviness of the jawline sagging of the chin skin

13 Zygomaticus M = Major, m = minor

14 Levator labii superioris
n = Levator labii superioris alaeque nasi

15 Orbicularis oculi

16 Depressor supercili

17 Corrugator

18 Procerus

19 Epicranius = Frontalis + Galea aponeurosis + Occcipitalis (not seen)

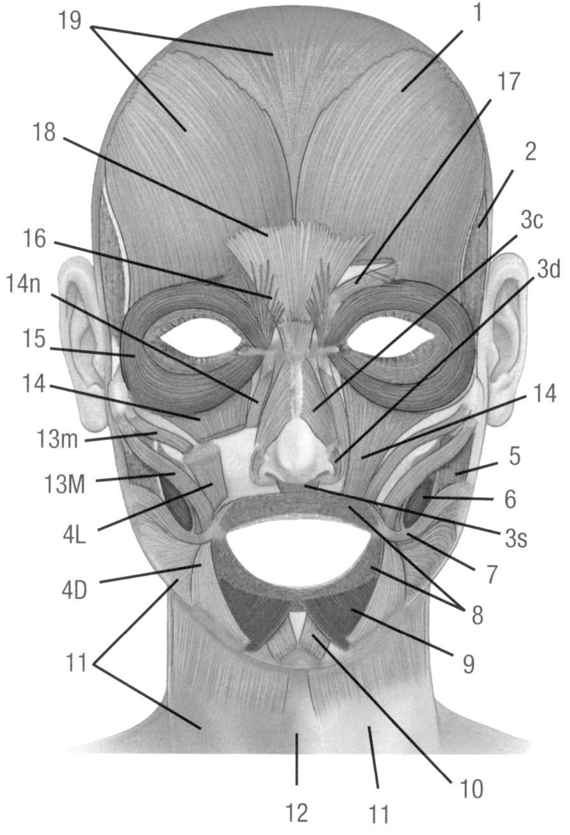
19
1
17
18
2
3c
16
3d
14n
15
14
14
13m
5
13M
6
4L
3s
7
4D
8
11
9
10
12
11

Muscles of the Face – Expression

Anterolateral view

Description: These muscles are often involved in cosmetic surgery and their function may be compromised by incisions at the level of the deep fascia.

1 Buccinator
2 Corrugator supercili
3 Depressor anguli Oris
4 Depressor labii inferioris, (overlying incisivus inf.)
5 Depressor septi
6 Frontalis (of occipitofrontalis)
7 Levator anguli oris (caninus),
8 Levator labii superioris
9 Levator labii superioris alaeque nasi (overlying Incisivus sup.)
10 Mentalis
11 Nasalis (compressor & dilator)
12 Orbicularis oculi
13 Orbicularis oris
14 Platysma
15 Procerus
16 Risorius
17 Zygomaticus major
18 Zygomaticus minor

NS facial N (CN VII) - supplies most of the muscles of the face
BS facial

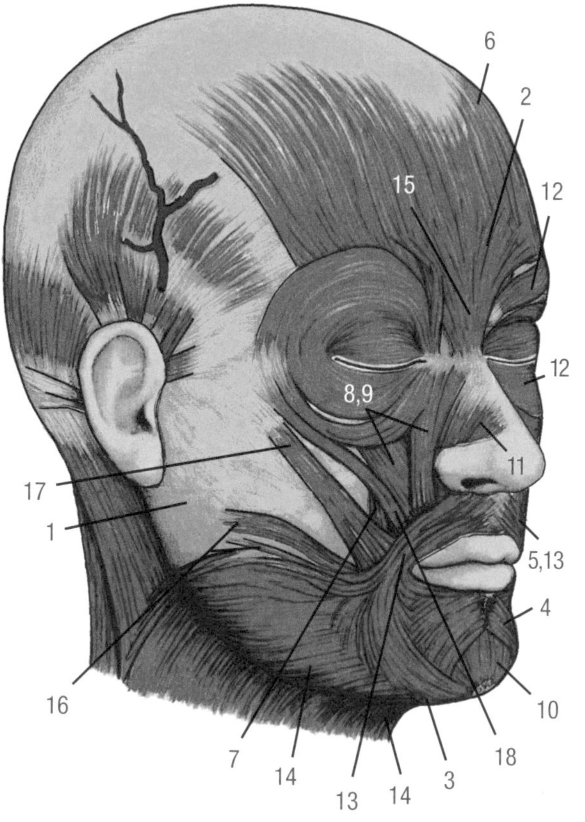
6
2
15
12
12
8,9
11
17
1
5,13
4
16
10
7
14
13
14
3
18

Mastication *Coronal section posterior view*

Primary movers of the Mandible + chewing and initiation of swallowing.

Muscles of mastication are all attached to the Mandible (Jaw bone) and are part of the Splanchnocranium. Those initiating swallowing move the food to the back of the throat & then into the oropharynx.

19 Masseter (F = Fascia)
20 Pterygoids Lateral (deep to Masseter)
21 Pterygoids Medial (deep to Buccinator)
22 Temporalis

NS trigeminal N –mandibular branch (CN V_3)
BS trigeminal and facial branches

Articulation & Swallowing

Primarily involved in speech and initiation of swallowing. They are often involved in "Stroke" patients affecting both speech and eating. *Not all demonstrated here.

31 Genioglossus
32 Geniohyoid
33 Styloglossus*
34 Hypoglossus
35 Stylohyoid*
36 Thyrohyoid*
37 Sternohyoid*
38 Sternothyroid*
39 Mylohyoid
40 Digastric*

NS hypoglossal (CN XII) and C1-3 of ansa cervicalis
BS facial a & branches

50 Mandibular sling = insertion raphe
51 Mandibular condyle
52 Interarticular disc of the TMJ
53 Sphenoid

* *See Muscles of the Hyoid.*

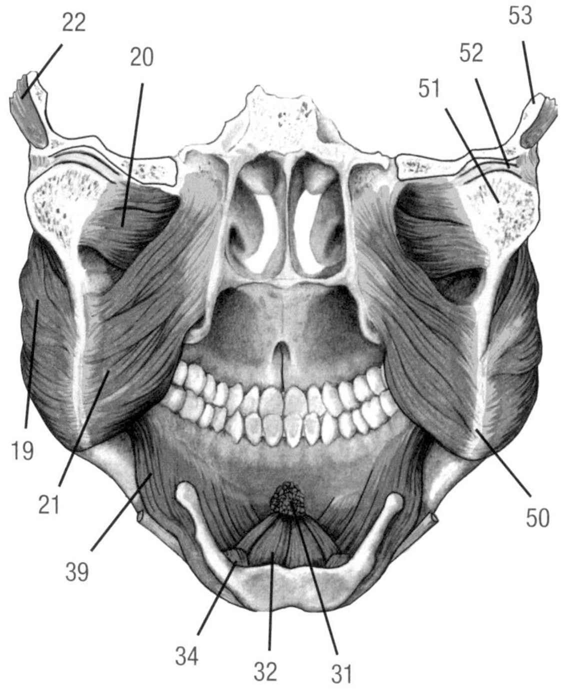
22
20
53
52
51
19
21
39
50
34
32
31

Muscles of Mastication – Chewing Masseter, Temporalis

Lateral view – Temporalis cut to show the medial Pterygoid

Description: Biting involves 2 muscles – Masseter & Temporalis and the teeth – Chewing involves 3 others the Buccinator & the Pterygoids and the Tongue.

There is a close association b/n these structures & the salivary glands.

1 Temporalis – attached to the conoid process of the Mandible (not shown)

2 Zygoma

3 Maxilla

4 Buccinator

5 incisor tooth

6 Masseter m

7 Sublingual salivary gland – smallest gland

8 Parotid gland - largest – most serous gland

9 Submandibular gland

10 angle of the jaw

11 medial pterygoid m

12 EAM

13 TMJ

for more details of the bones & muscles see **the A to Z of the Head & Neck muscles & bones (note some texts use the terms internal and external Pterygoids to represent the medial and lateral respectively)*

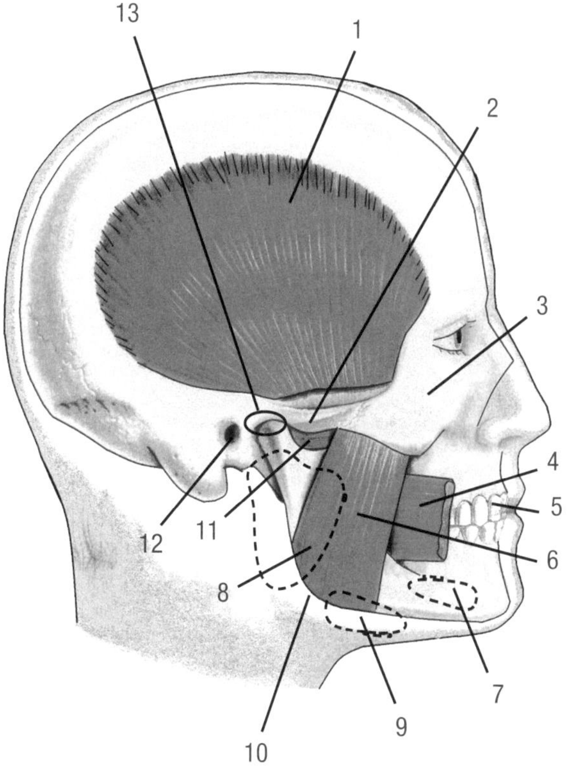
13
1
2
3
4
5
6
7
8
9
10
11
12

Muscles of the Hyoid bone & Thyroid cartilage (Larynx)

The Hyoid bone and the Larynx hang b/n the SUPRA-HYOID and INFRAHYOID muscles

They move with swallowing, breathing and speech

SWALLOWING cannot commence w/o the Mandible being fixed

It cannot continue w/o the Sternum and Clavicle being fixed to allow for the Hyoid to be depressed

Arrows show the directions of the muscles

These muscles determine the chin line and are involved in cosmetic surgery – Several muscles rely on tendinous slings and have two bellies to function.

Elevator Muscles

1 Palatoglossus
2 Stylopharyngeus
3 Thyrohyoid
4 Pharyngeal constrictors
5 Stylohyoid
6 Geniohyoid
7 Digastric m this muscle has 2 bellies ant & post
8 Mylohyoid

Depressor Muscles

9 Sternohyoid
10 Omohyoid
11 Sternothyroid
3 Thyrohyoid (both functions)

NS ansa cervicalis C1-3
BS facial and thyroid vessels

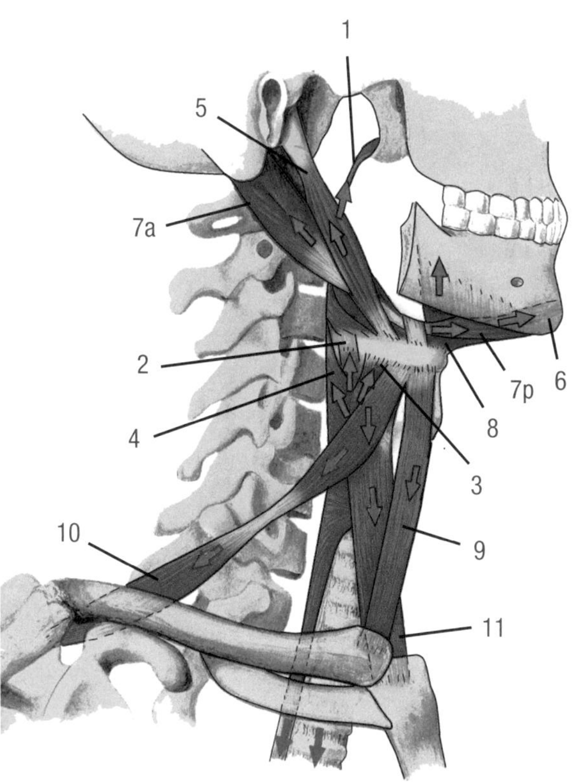
1
5
7a
2
4
10
7p
6
8
3
9
11

Muscles of the Pharynx

Lateral

Description: The space b/n the mouth and oesophagus – a modified muscular tube directing the food bolus to the GIT.

Lifting the Pharynx closes the auditory tube and nasopharynx (10,11) food moves to the back of the throat – swallowing begins coordinated by the constrictors (1). It is supported by ligs (3,12) & muscles (2).

NS facial, maxillary
BS CN X – vagus, branches of ansa cervicalis (C1-3)

1 Pharyngeal constrictors m
  i = inferior
  m = middle
  s = superior
2 Stylopharyngeus m
3 Stylohyoid lig
4 Thyroid cartilage
5 Thyrohyoid membrane
6 Hyoid bone
7 Mylohyoid m
8 Mandible
9 Buccinator m
10 Palatopharyngeus m
11 Salpingopharyngeus m
12 Cricothyroid m
13 Oesophagus
14 Trachea

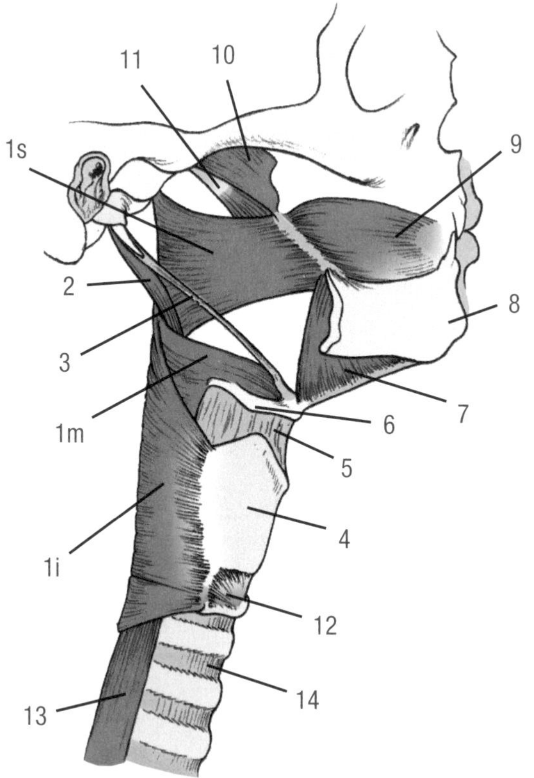
11
10
1s
9
2
8
3
7
6
1m
5
4
1i
12
14
13

Muscles of the Tongue – overview

coronal

sagittal

Description: The tongue is a "bag of muscles"with a fixed pharyngeal root and free oral tip / apex. Muscle which move it from w/in - intrinsic and those which change its position from w/out are extrinsic.

Extrinsic

Genioglossus (4) - attaches to the Hyoid, Pharyngeal constrictors, Hypoglossus and intrinsic Lingualis muscles to protrude tongue (poke out the tongue) depress the centre and raise the sides (make a tunnel with the tongue)

Hyoglossus (3) - attaches to the front and horns of the Hyoid, side of the tongue and intrinsic Lingualis muscles in order to depress the tongue (as in say AHHHHH…)

Palatoglossus (5) – attached to the palatine aponeurosis & blends with the lateral Linguali muscles

Styloglossus (2) - attaches to the styloid process, and blends with the Hypoglossus, Stylohyoid

Intrinsic

Linguali muscles (1)- superior, inferior, transverse and vertical

attach w/in the tongue to change its shape for speech, in mastication and swallowing

NS lingual, sublingual and hypoglossal (CN XII) Ns
BS lingual, sublingual and external carotid

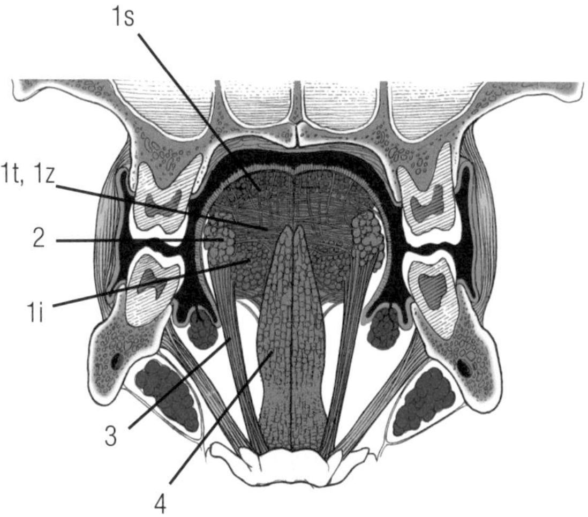

1s
1t, 1z
2
1i
3
4

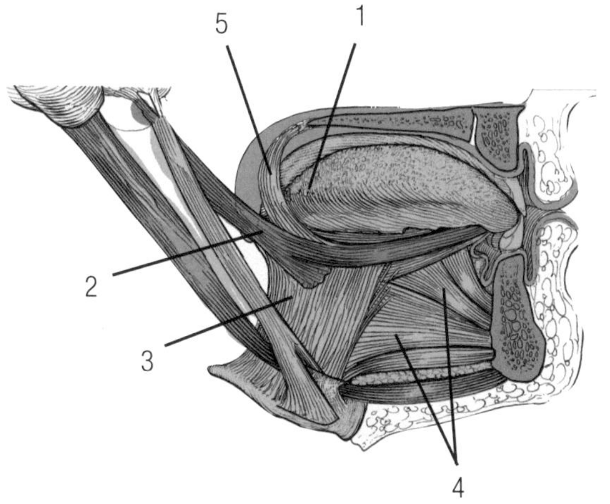

Examination of Skeletal Muscles - major groups

note detailed examinations of individual muscles are listed in ***The A to Z of Sensory and Muscles testing*** and ***The A to Z of the Peripheral Nerves*** and in ***The A to Z of Bone and Joint Failure,*** as well as general testing listed after each muscle in the text. ROM and a selection of strength tests of major movements are included here

Hx - questions for individual joint examination

1. functional limitation
2. SS - limited to one or more joints
3. onset- acute - related to a specific incident
   - chronic - slow progressive increase of pain or reduced ROM
4. description of the causative agent if known e.g. accident
5. any prior MSS history of that joint or others
6. Systemic problems

Ex - for participation in sport / training activities MSS

for this examination unless otherwise indicated the patient standing - facing the clinician in the anatomical position - *included are several tests with the patient in alternative positions for specific testing*

CERVICAL SPINE / NECK - ROM tests the following groups of muscles

Scalenes / Colles / Trapezius upper fibres / Cervicis regions of ES and deep muscles of the VC / Sternocleidomastoid

patient looks at the roof ± R	extension
patient looks at the floor ± R	flexion
patient looks over each shoulder ± R	horizontal rotation
head bends towards the shoulder - sideways ± R (shoulders kept still)	lateral flexion

SHOULDER (SCAPULA) - ROM tests the following groups of muscles

Levator Scapulae / Rhomboids / Serratus Anterior / Spinati muscles / Trapezius / Deltoid

observe symmetry of shoulder particularly the Acromioclavicular jt

shrug shoulders ± R	elevation
drop shoulders	depression
straighten shoulders - trying to meet shoulder blades	lateral rotation
contract shoulders – withdrawing chest	medial rotation
abduct shoulders to 90° (flexed arm) ± R	abduction

Strength tests - Shoulder

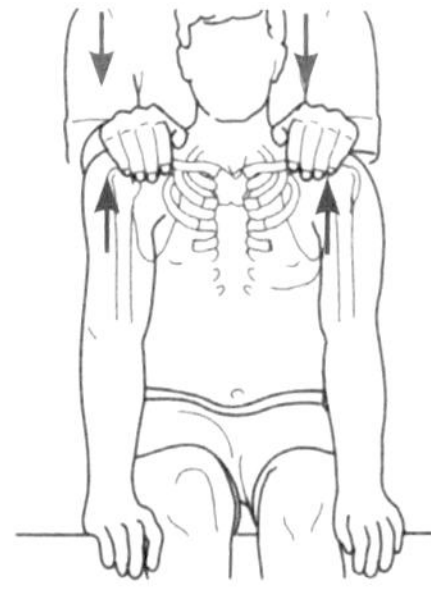

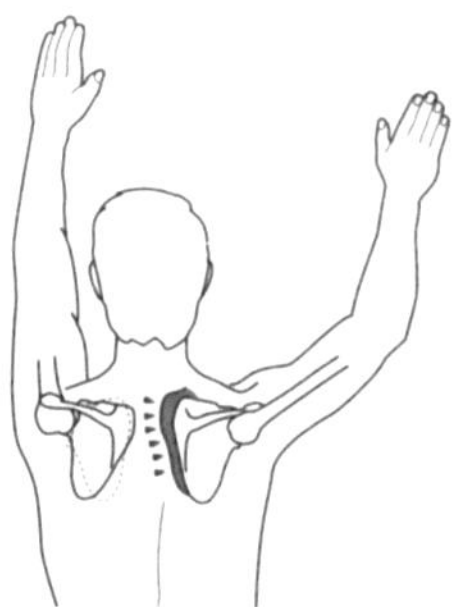

SHOULDER + ARM – ROM tests the following groups of muscles

Pectorals / Latisimus Dorsi / Trapezius / Scapular muscles

scratch back with each hand from over and under the shoulder <u>or</u> have hands meet at the back from over and under the shoulder	external rotation + abduction internal rotation + adduction
move extended abducted arms as high as possible ± R	vertical adduction
move extended abducted arms into the sagittal plane ± R	horizontal adduction
move extended abducted arms out of the sagittal plane ± R	horizontal abduction
with bent arms keep them close to the body against R	adduction

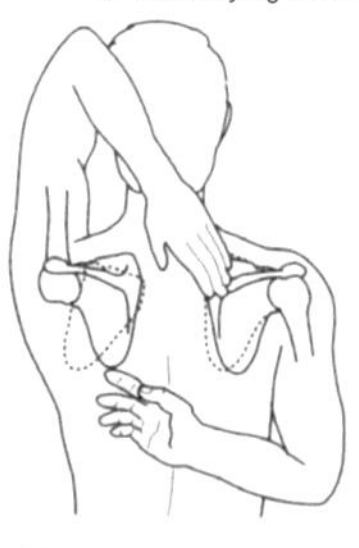

full ROM of the shoulder, scapula and upper limb

UPPER LIMB + HAND - ROM tests the following groups of muscles

Brachii muscles / Brachioradialis / Flexors & Extensors of upper limb, hand & digits / Supinators / Pronators / Carpi muscles / Intrinsic muscles of the hand

flex/extend elbows ± R	
turn wrist in and out ± R	pronation/supination
bend and straighten wrist ± R	flexion/extension
move extended wrist towards the body ± R	ulnar deviation = medial flexion
move extended wrist away from the body ± R	radial deviation = lateral flexion
spread extended fingers ± R	abduction
close extended open fingers ± R	adduction
oppose fingers and thumb	opposition
make a fist ± R	flexion
extend hand and fingers ± R	extension

Testing elbow extension / flexion

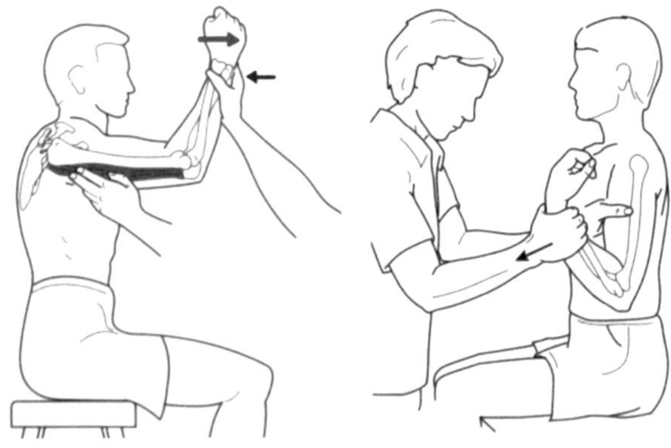

Forearm Testing pronation and supination

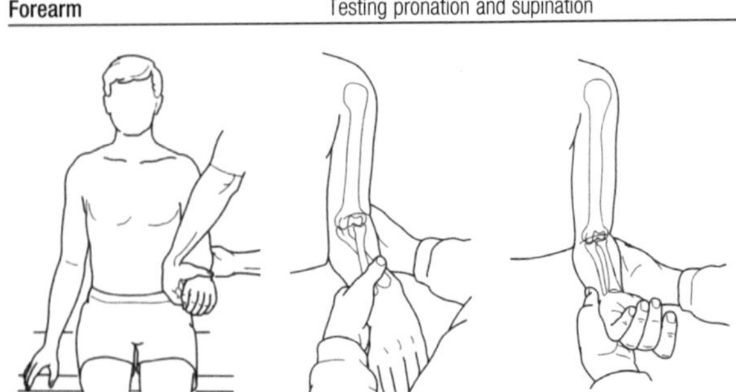

Wrist testing extension flexion

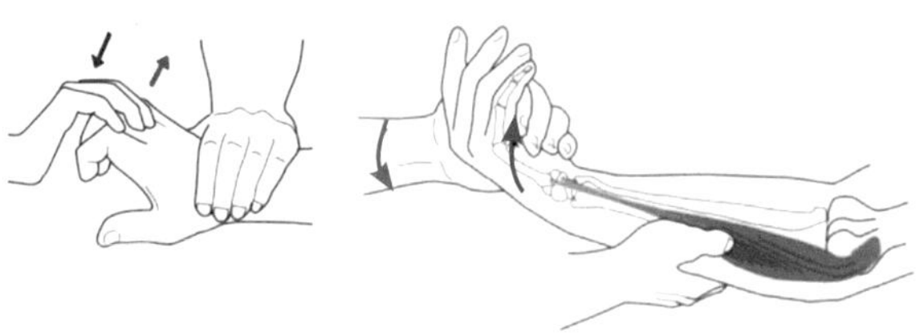

Fist

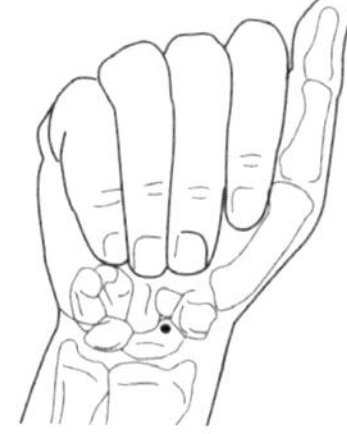

note the normal fist has all fingers pointing to the scaphoid tubercle normal flaxion of the IP joints

Thumb thumb adduction opposition

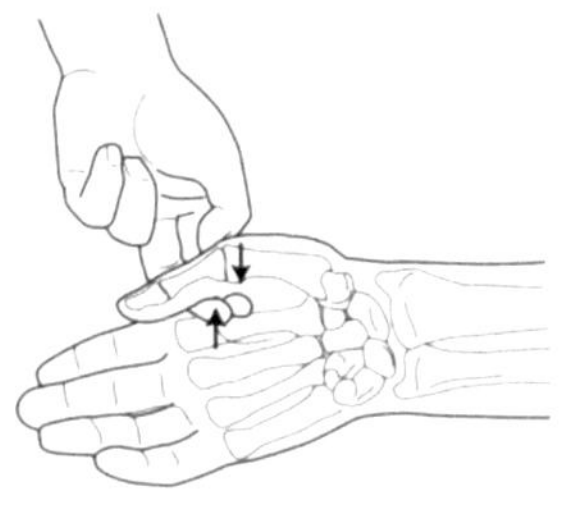

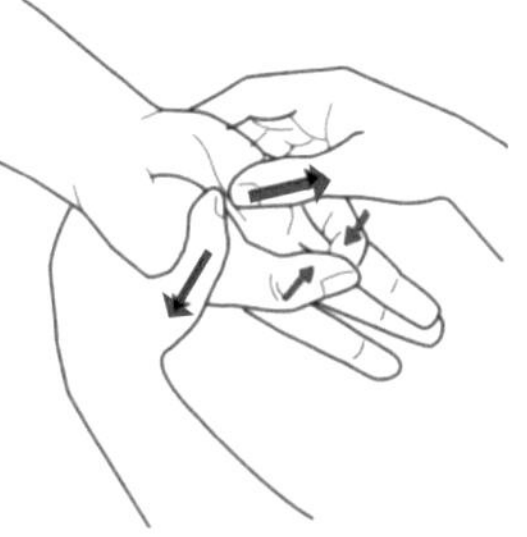

BACK ABDOMEN – ROM tests the following groups of muscles

ES, deep muscles of the back, Latissimus Dorsi, Quadratus Lumborum, Obliques, Gluteal muscles, Rectus Abdominus

observe posture, shoulder and neck symmetry, spinal curvature	
observe for balance on one leg	
bend from side to side while facing the front	lateral flexion
bend back as far as possible	hyperextension
twist from the hips to the left & right	rotation
supine patient - touch toes and back (back/abdomen)	extension/flexion

Strength tests - Abdomen

testing abdominal flexion - abdominal rotation

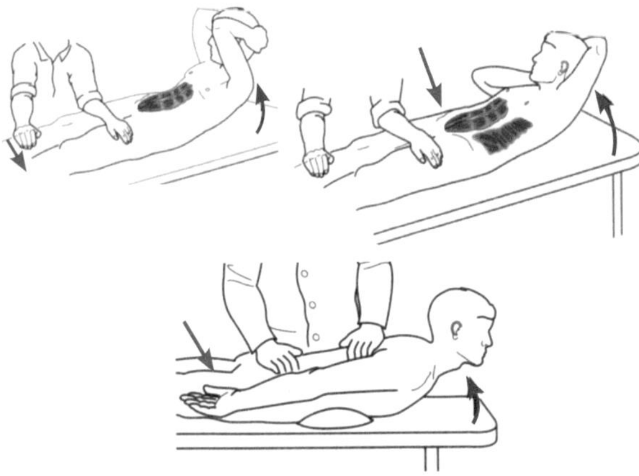

HIP + THIGH - ROM tests the following muscles

Gluteal muscles / Iliopsoas / Obturators / Quadriceps / Hamstrings / Adductors / Abductors

observe symmetry of the hips and stance	
turn leg inwards/outwards	medial/lateral rotation
standing patient - touch toes with straight legs	extension/flexion (back) & hamstring tightness
lift the extended leg forwards/backwards	flexion/extension (hip)
lift the extended leg sideways	lateral flexion (hip)
with the sitting patient keep legs together against R	adduction

Hip

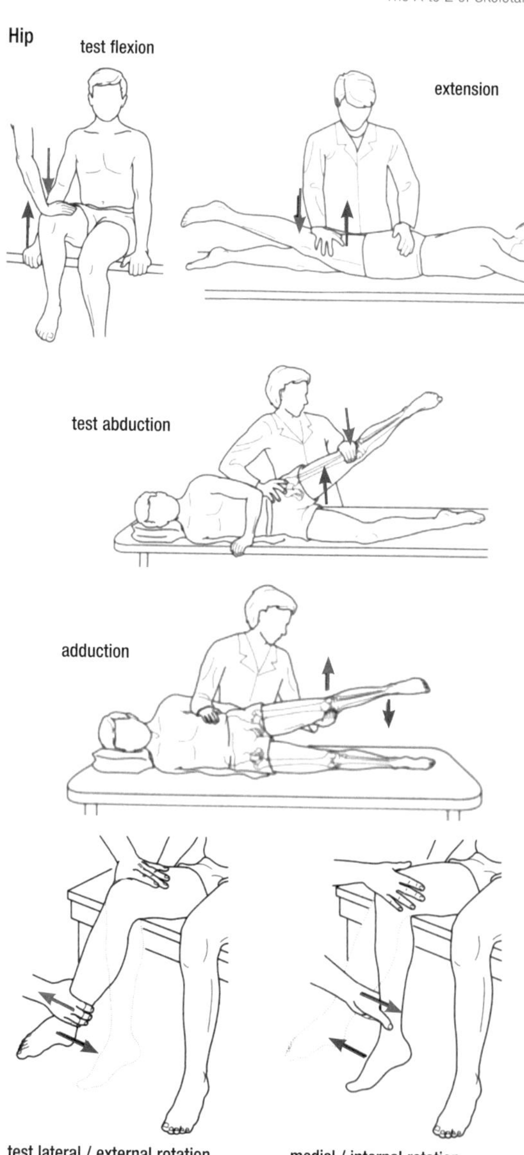
test flexion
extension
test abduction
adduction
test lateral / external rotation
medial / internal rotation

LOWER LIMB + KNEE + ANKLE + FOOT + TOES – ROM tests the following groups of muscles

Gluteal muscles / Iliopsoas / Quadriceps / Hamstrings / Adductors / Abductors / Peroneal muscles / Soleus / Intrinsic muscles of the foot

observe for knee & ankle symmetry - looking for effusions &/or deformities

bend and straighten legs with erect posture	flexion/extension (knee & ankle)
spread toes	abduction (toes)
point toes	plantar flexion (ankle)
duckwalk with buttocks on heals - this tests all	lower limb and hip ROM
point feet outwards/inwards	eversion/inversion (foot)

Strength tests - Knee

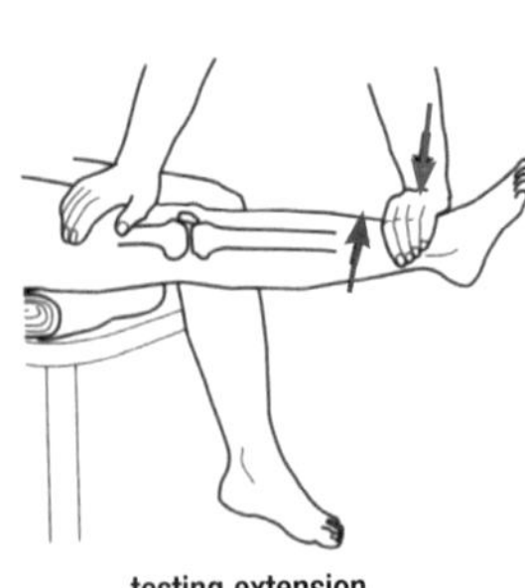

testing extension

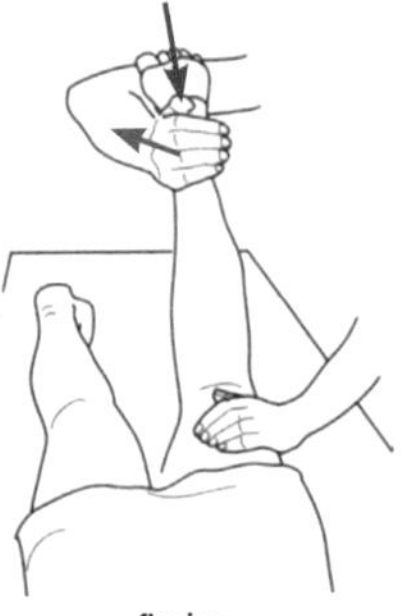

flexion

Ankle

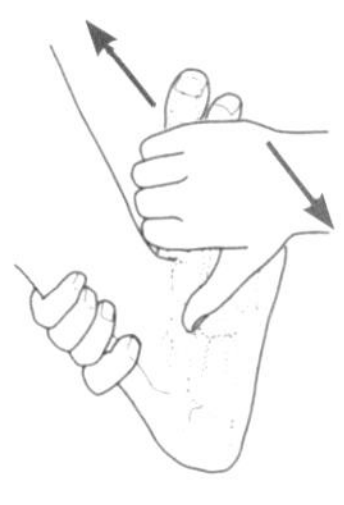

testing dorsiflexion

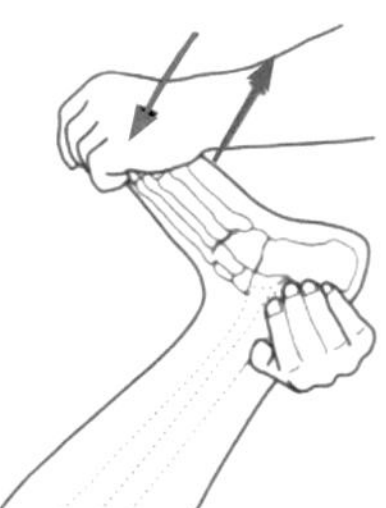

plantar flexion

Toes

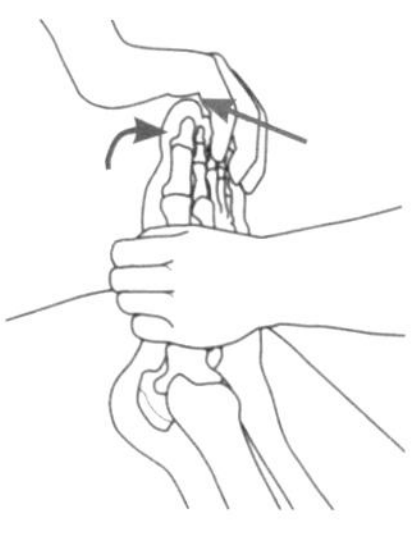

testing extension

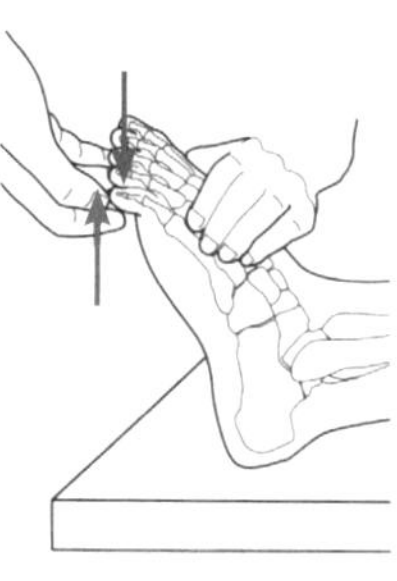

flexion

Skeletal Muscle Groupings

Skeletal Muscle Groups

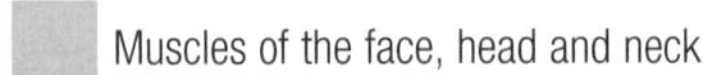
Muscles of the face, head and neck

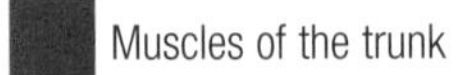
Muscles of the trunk

Muscles of the back and spine

Muscles of the chest, shoulder, forearm and hand

Muscles of the hip, thigh, leg and foot

Muscles of the pelvis and perineum

Please use this colour coding as a guide only for muscle positions and placements; double colour codes may be used for muscles which cover 2 anatomical regions.

Skeletal Muscle Groupings

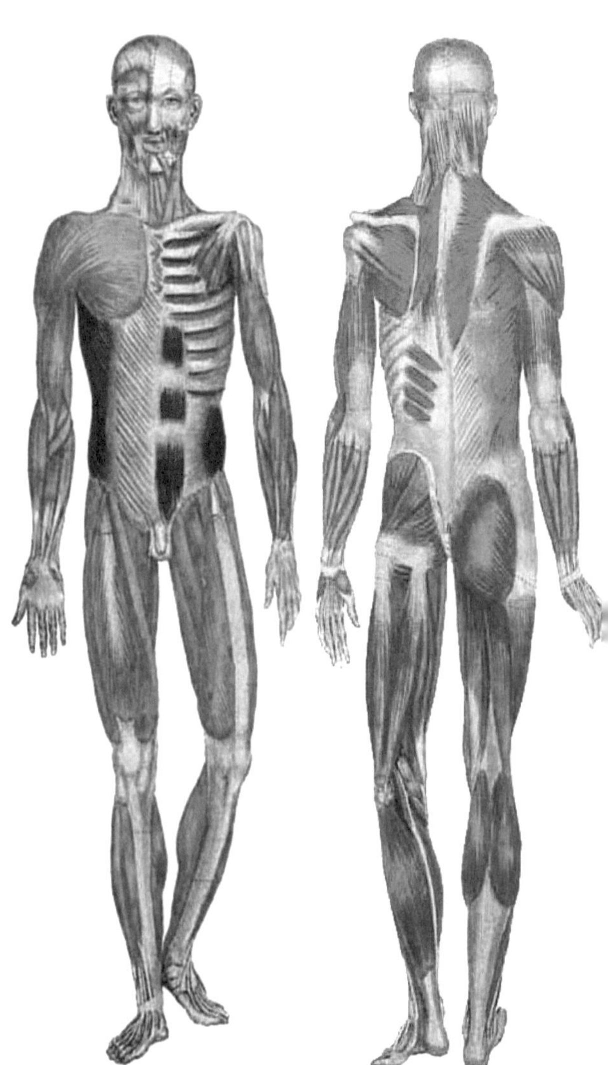

Index of Muscles

- Muscles of the hip, thigh leg and foot
- Muscles of the chest, shoulder, forearm and hand
- Muscles of the face, head and neck
- Muscles of the trunk
- Muscles of the back and spine
- Muscles of the pelvis and perineum

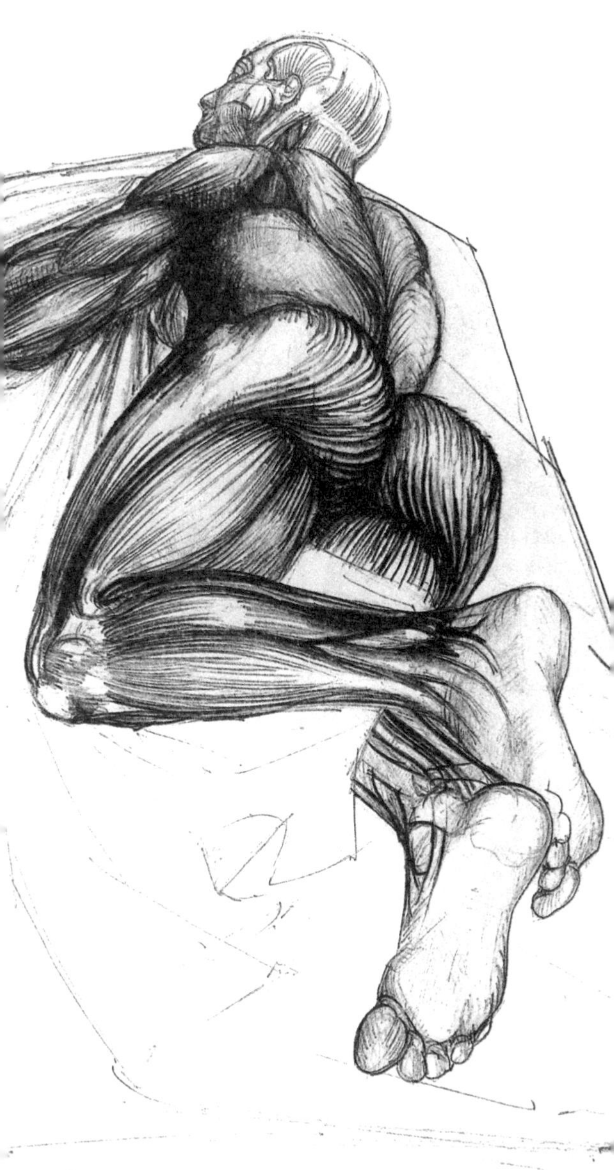

Abductor Digiti Minimi (foot)

most superficial layer of the sole of the foot

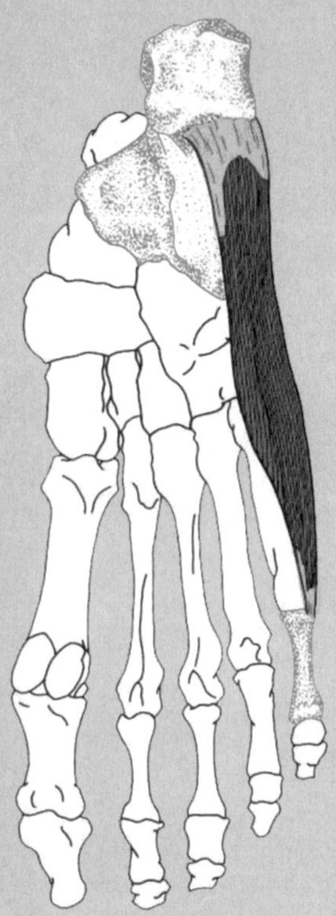

O - medial & lateral process of Calcaneal tuberosity
  - Plantar Aponeurosis
I - lateral base Phalanx 1 Digit 5
A - abduction
NS - lateral plantar N (L4-5)
BS - lateral plantar
T - abduction against R

Abductor Digiti Minimi (hand)

Hypothenar eminence

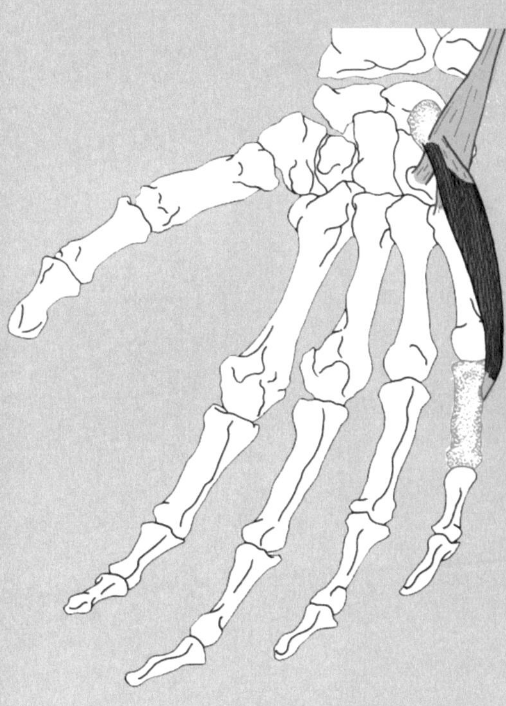

O - Pisiform
    - tendon of Flexor Carpi Ulnaris
I - ulnar side Phalanx 1 Digit 5
A - abduction
NS - ulnar N (C8-T1)
BS - ulnar
T - abduction against R

Abductor Hallicus

most superficial layer of the sole of the foot

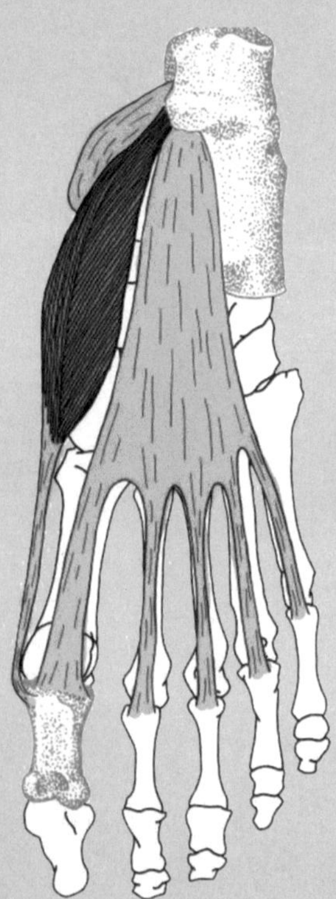

O - medial process of Calcaneal tuberosity
- Plantar Aponeurosis / Flexor Retinaculum

I - medial base Phalanx 1 Digit 1

A - abduction

NS - medial plantar N (L4-5)

BS - medial plantar

T - abduction against R

Abductor Pollicus Brevis
part of the thenar eminence

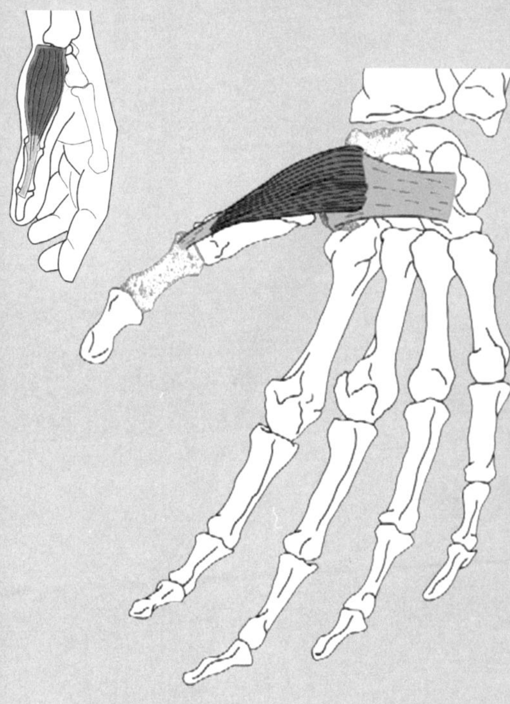

O - ridge of Trapezium
- Flexor Retinaculum
- Scaphoid

I - lateral Phalanx 1 Digit 1
A - abduction / anterior movement of thumb
NS - median N (C7-T1)
BS - radial
T - abduction against R - at MCP

Abductor Pollicus Longus

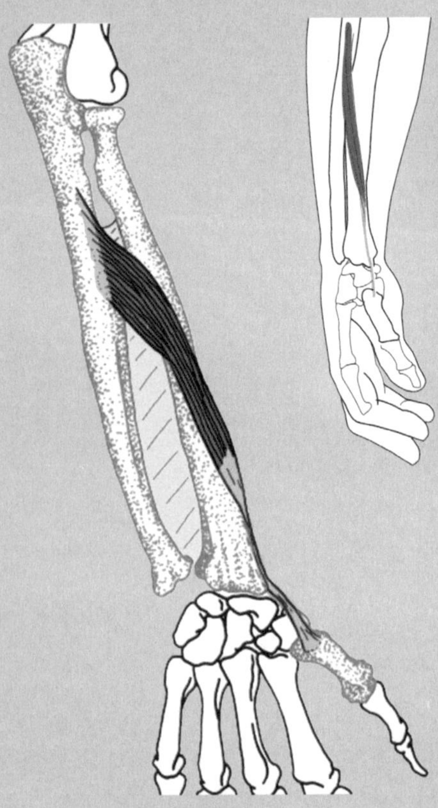

O - posterior Radius
- posterior Ulna
- interosseus membrane

I - lateral base of MC 1

A - abduction of hand and thumb

NS - radial N (C6-7)

BS - radial / ulnar

T - abduction against R - at MCP

Adductor Brevis
part of the medial compartment of the thigh

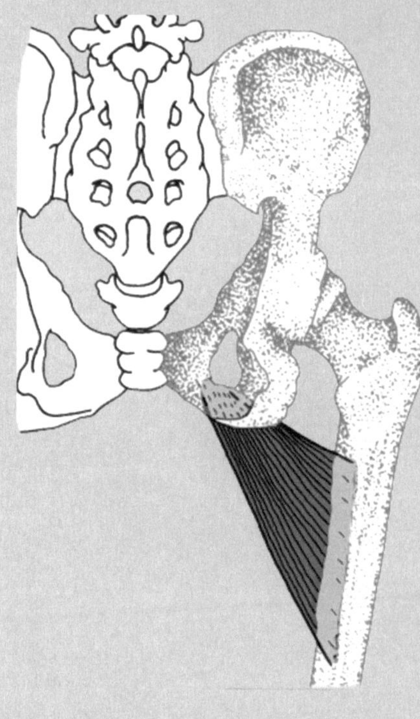

O - inferior pubic ramis of hip
I - upper medial lip of linea aspera (Femur)
A - adduction / hip flexion
NS - obturator N (L2-4)
BS - obturator
T - adduct legs against R in the supine patient

Adductor Hallicus

part of the third layer of the sole of the foot

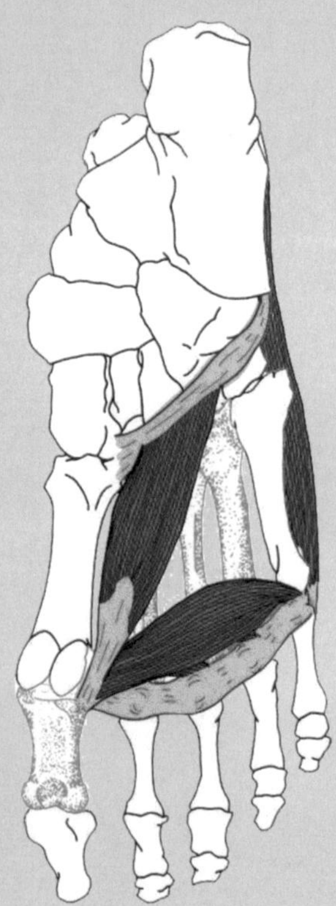

O - oblique head - base MTs 2-4
- transverse head - sheath/tendon of Peroneus Longus
- plantar MCPs of Digits 3-5

I - lateral base of Phalanx 1 Digit 1

A - adduction

NS - lateral plantar N (deep branch) (L4-5)

BS - 1st plantar MT

T - separate big toe against R

Adductor Longus

part of the medial compartment of the thigh

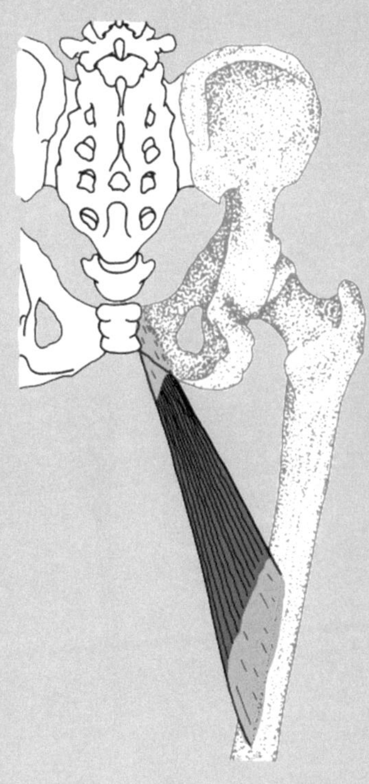

O - pubic symphysis of hip
I - middle medial lip of linea aspera (Femur)
A - adduction / hip flexion
NS - obturator N (L2-4)
BS - obturator
T - adduct legs against R in the supine patient

Adductor Magnus

part of the medial compartment of the thigh

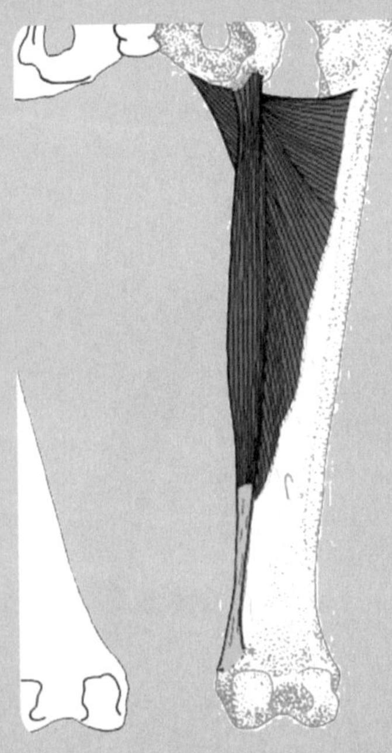

O - pubic symphysis, ischeal ramus of hip
I - linea aspera, adductor tubercle (Femur)
A - adduction / hip flexion & extension
NS - obturator N + sciatic N (L2-4)
BS - obturator, medial circumflex, femoral
T - adduct legs against R in the supine patient

Adductor Pollicus

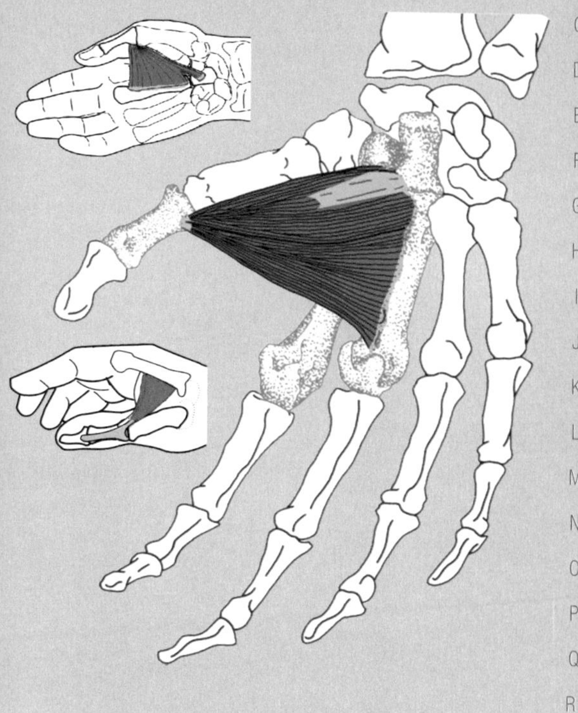

O - transverse head of MC 3
- Capitate (oblique head)
- Trapezium
- Trapezoid

I - lateral base of Phalanx 1 Digit 1

A - adduction of thumb

NS - ulnar N (deep branch) (C8-T1)

BS - deep palmar arch

T - close hand against R to the thumb

Anconeus

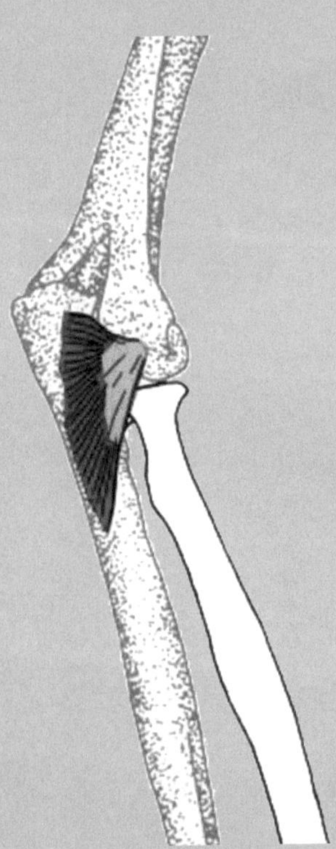

O - posterior lateral condyle - Capitulum (Humerus)
I - posterior Olecranon process (Ulna)
A - elbow extension
NS - radial N (C7-8)
BS - brachial (deep branch)
T - extend elbow against R

Aryepiglotticus - *see Muscles of the Larynx*

Arytenoids - Oblique, Transverse - *see Muscles of the Larynx*

Auricularis

anterior, superior, posterior
= Extrinsic muscles of the Ear (present in 30%)

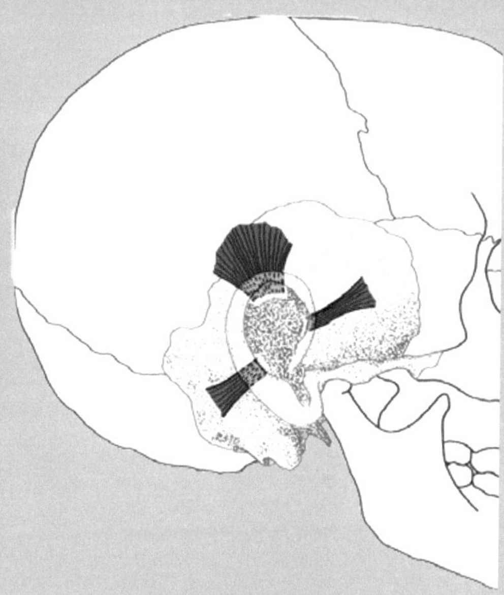

O - ant. Epicranial Aponeurosis
- post. Mastoid process of Temporalis
- sup. Epicranial Aponeurosis

I - ant. root of Auricle
- post. root of Auricle
- sup. root of Auricle

A - moves ear Pinna

NS - facial N (CN VII)

BS - facial / temporal

T - present if there is movement of the ear

Biceps Brachii

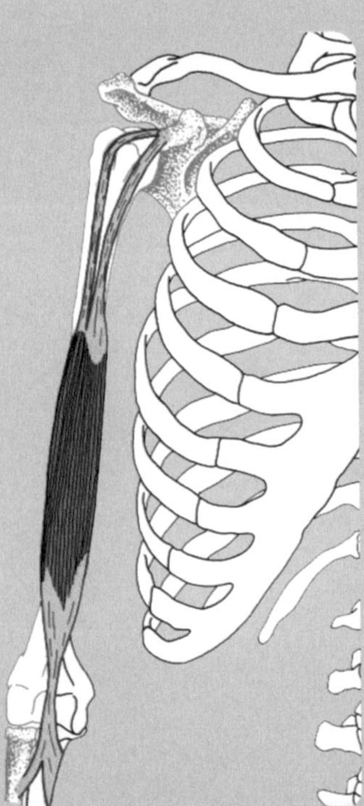

O - long head superior lip of Glenoid fossa (Scapula)
- short head Coracoid process (Scapula)

I - tuberosity (Radius)

A - flexion (shoulder & elbow)
- supination (hand & forearm)

NS - musculocutaneous N (C5-6)

BS - brachial (deep branch)

T - flex elbow against R - elbow placed on table at 90º

Biceps Femoris

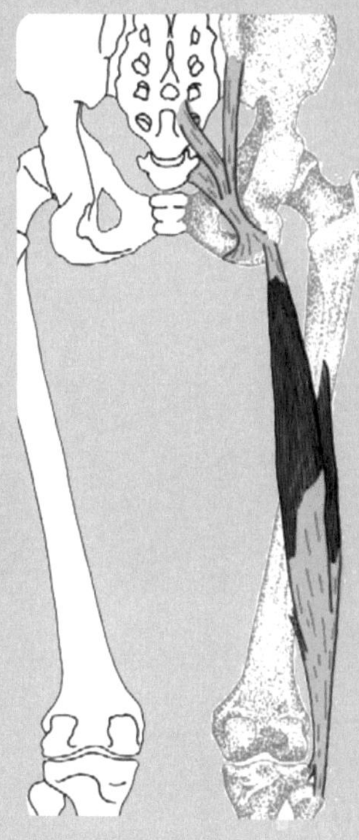

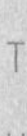

O - ischeal tuberosity (hip)
   - linea aspera (Femur)
I - head of Fibula
A - extension (hip)
   - flexion (knee)
   - rotation (flexed knee)
NS - sciatic N (L5-S2)
BS - deep femoral
   - popliteal
T - extend hip against R
   - flex knee against R - in the prone patient

Brachialis

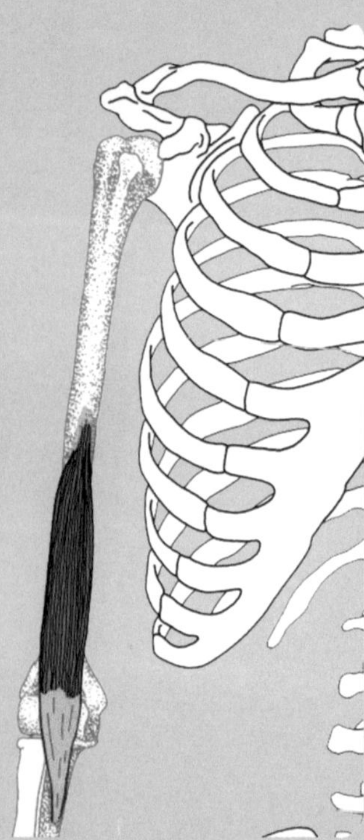

O - lower ½ of the Humerus
I - coronoid process (Ulna)
A - flexion (elbow)
NS - musculocutaneous N (C5-6)
BS - brachial (deep branch)
- radial recurrent
T - flex elbow against R - elbow placed on table at 90°

Brachioradialis

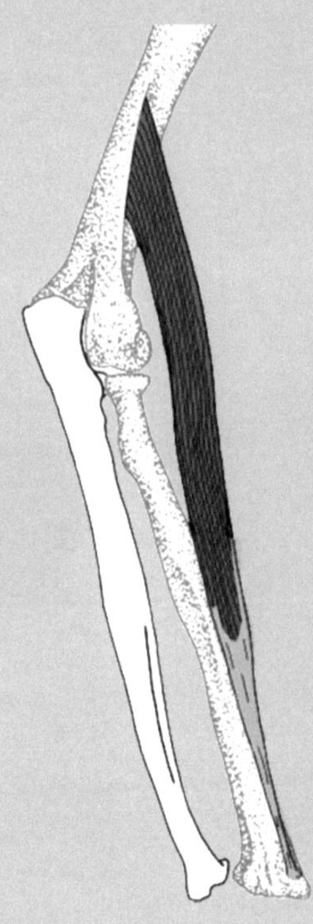

O - lateral supracondylar ridge (Humerus)
I - styloid process (Radius)
A - flexion (elbow)
- pronation (forearm)
NS - radial N (C5-6)
BS - radial recurrent
T - flex elbow against R - elbow placed on table at 90º

Buccinator
part of the muscles of mastication

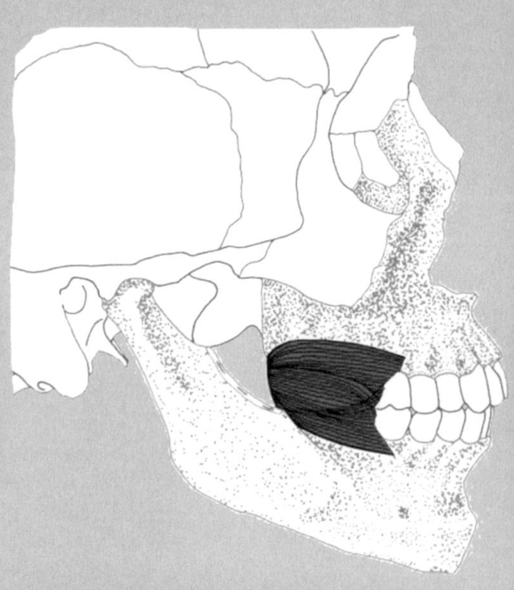

O - lateral – outer surface of alveolar process of Maxilla
  - lateral surface (Mandible)
I - deep part of the muscles of the lips
  - deep fascia of the face
A - compresses cheeks
  - draws down angle of the mouth
NS - facial N (CN VII)
BS - facial
T - ask patient to blow as if playing the saxaphone.

Bulbospongiosus - *see Muscles of the Perineum*
Ciliaris - *see Muscles of the Eye*

Coccygeus = Ischeococcygeus - *see the muscles of the Perineum*

Coracobrachialis

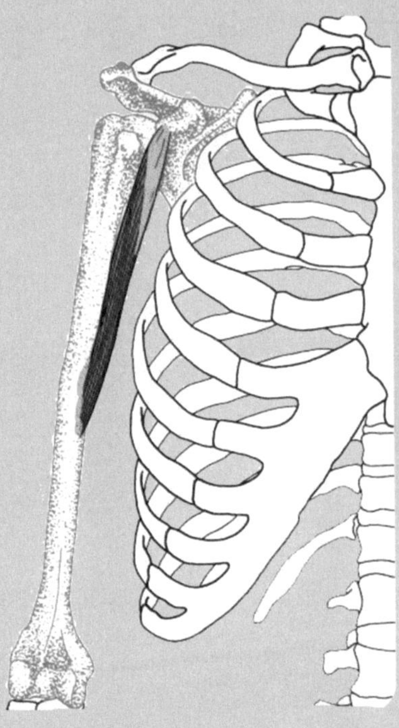

O - corocoid process (Scapula)
I - midshaft of the Humerus
A - adduction (arm & shoulder)
NS - musculocutaneous N (C6-7)
BS - brachial
T - moving extended arm supported on a table to the midline against R

Corrugator Supercilii

part of the muscles of facial expression

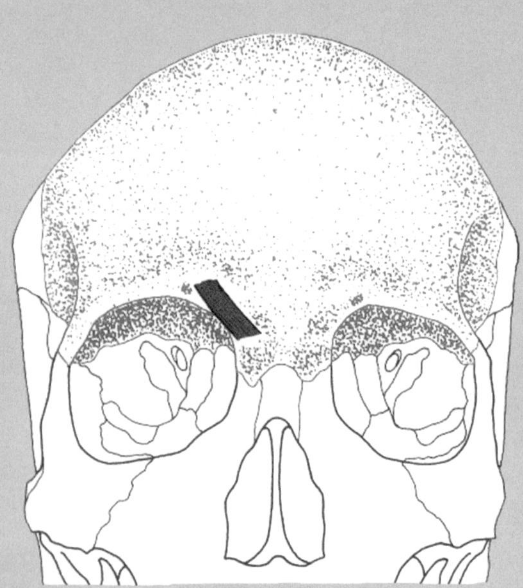

O - glabella (Frontalis)
- medial suprorbital margin (Frontalis)

I - deep fascia of the skin in the midpoint of the orbital arch

A - pulls brows down and medially frowning

NS - facial N, supraorbital supratrochlear branches (CN VII)

BS - facial opthalmic artery

T - ability to wrinkle brow

Cremaster
part of the muscles of the perineum

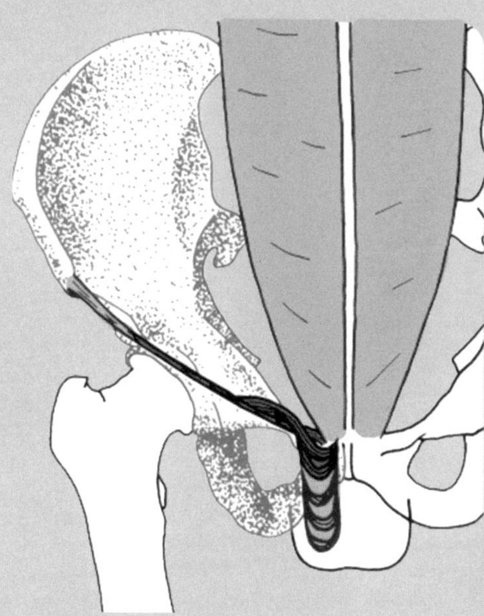

O - inguinal ligament
I - pubic tubercle (hip)
A - pulls testis to the body /regulates temperature of the testis
NS - genitofemoral, genital branch (L1-2)
BS - genitofemoral, genital branch
T - testis jumps up when the thigh is stroked
  - labia majora twitches

Deltoid

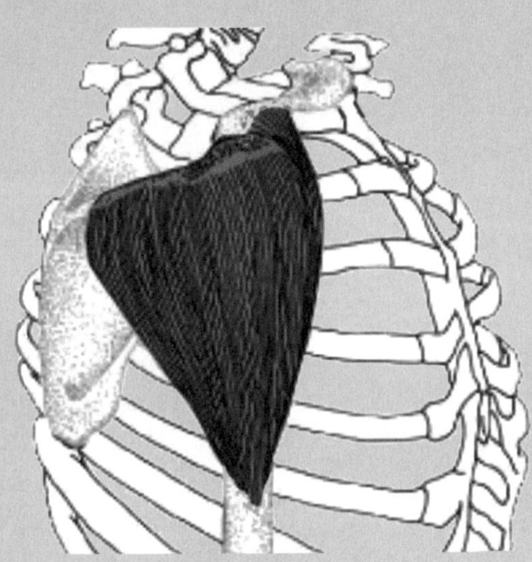

O - lateral 1/3 of anterior surface of Clavicle
- acromion process (Scapula)
- posterior spine (Scapula)

I - deltoid tuberosity (Humerus)

A - <u>anterior</u> - shoulder flexion, adduction, medial rotation abduction >90°, horizontal swing to midline
- middle - shoulder abduction >90°
- posterior - shoulder extension, adduction, lateral rotation abduction >90° horizontal swing to midline,

NS - axillary N (C5-6)

BS - thoracoacromial

T - moving shoulder in most directions against R
- the supine patient will eliminate the influence of gravity

Depressor Anguli Oris
part of the muscles of facial expression

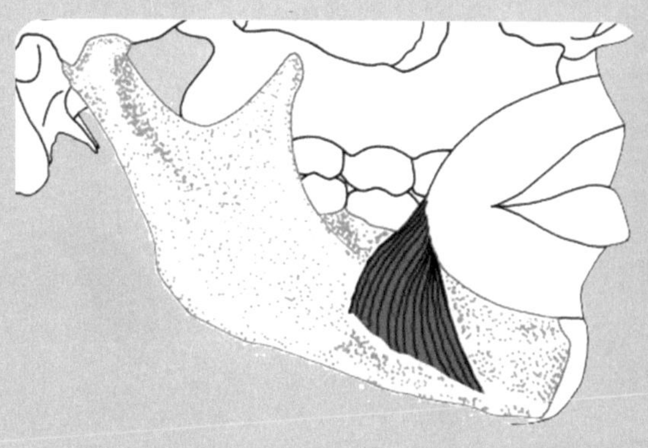

O - oblique lines (Mandible)
I - deep fascia - at the corner of the lips
A - turns the corners of the lips down as in frowning
NS - facial N, mandibular branch (CN VII)
BS - facial - maxillary branch + inferior labial branch
T - ability to turn down the corners of the mouth as in frowning

Depressor Labii Inferioris

part of the muscles of facial expression

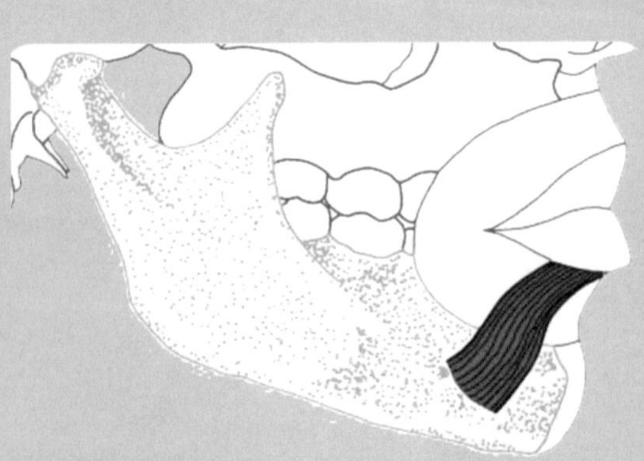

O - anterior-medial surfaces of Mandible
I - deep fascia medial to the corners of the lips
A - pulls lips down and back (with Platysma)
NS - facial N, superior buccal & mandibular branches (CN VII)
BS - facial - labial branches
T - ability to draw back lips and tighten neck (Platysma)

Depressor Septi
part of the muscles of facial expression

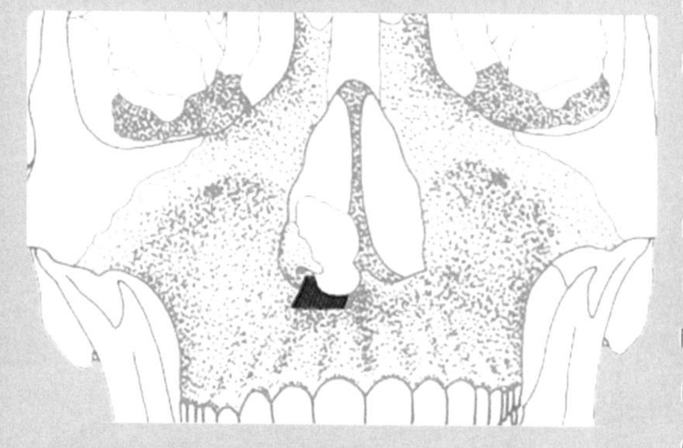

O - anterior - medial surfaces of Maxilla
I - deep fascia at the base of the nose
A - pulls nostrils inwards and lips up
NS - facial N, maxillary branch (CN VII)
BS - facial - maxillary, superior buccal branches
T - ask patient to wrinkle nose

Diaphragm

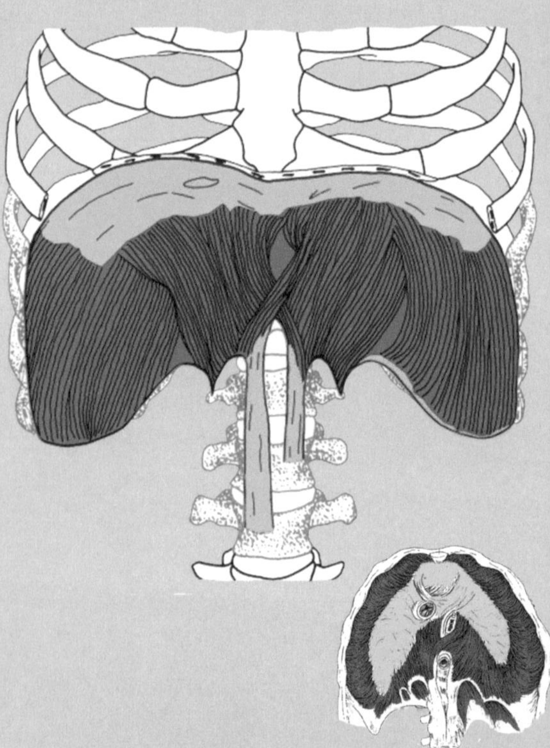

O - xiphoid process (Sternum)
- ribs 7-12
- lumbar vertebrae L1-2

I - central tendon

A - forced inspiration - pulls down central tendon and expands volume

NS - phrenic (C3-5)
- accessary phrenic, cervical plexus

BS - superior, inferior phrenic, mamillary & long thoracic

T - ask patient to force inspiration and note abdomen increase

Digastricus
part of the muscles of the Hyoid
(anterior neck 2 muscle bellies passing through a fibrous loop)

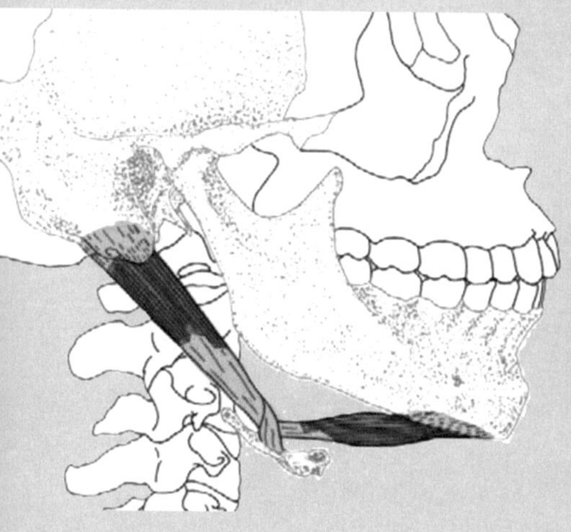

O - <u>anterior</u> - inner side (lingular) of jaw (Mandible)
- <u>posterior</u> - mastoid notch (Temporal bone)

I - slides through the Hyoid tendon / ligament

A - elevates, retracts and protracts Hyoid
- depresses Mandible

NS - <u>anterior</u> - trigeminal N (CN V)
- <u>posterior</u> - facial N (CN VII)

BS - facial mandibular branch
- superior cervical

T - open jaw against R
- note movement of Hyoid on swallowing

Dorsal Interossei (foot)

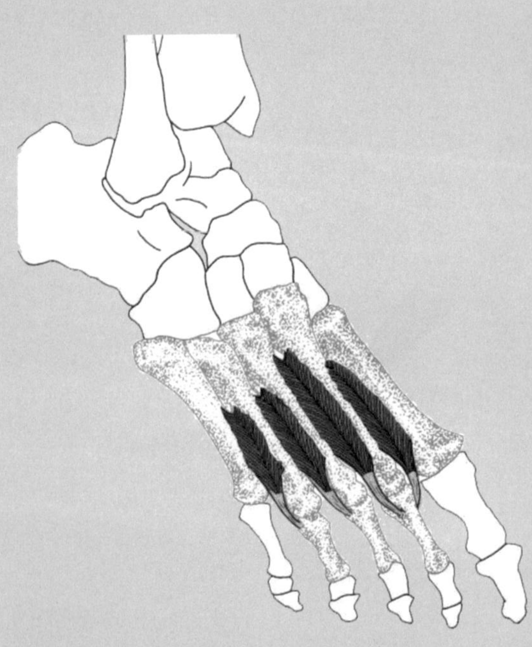

O - 2 heads to adjacent MTs 2-5
I - base Phalanx 1 Digits 2-5
A - abduction
NS - lateral plantar (superficial peroneal) (L4-S2)
BS - lateral plantar

Dorsal Interossei (hand)

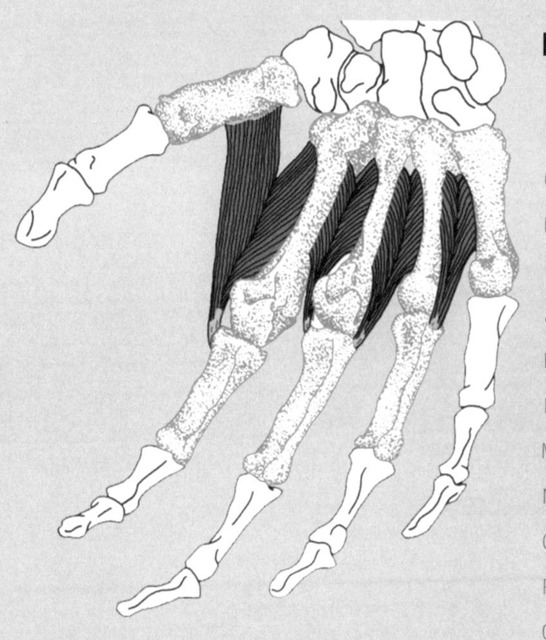

O - 2 heads to adjacent MCs 2-5
I - base Phalanx 1 Digits 2-5
A - abduction of fingers from and axis through middle finger
- flexion of proximal PIPs
- extension of middle and distal PIPs (fingers in a tent)
NS - ulnar N (C8-T1)
BS - deep palmer arch
T - open fingers against R
- straighten 1st jt of fingers and straighten out their ends

Epicranius = Frontalis + Occipitalis = Occipito-Frontalis

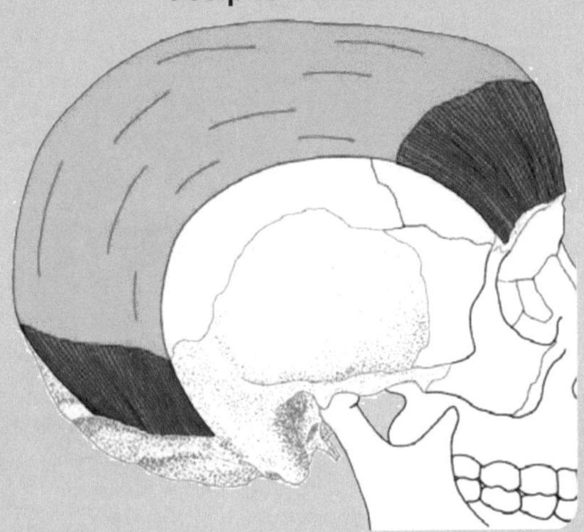

Frontalis

O - skull aponeurosis
I - superficial fascia superior to brow
A - raises eyebrows / wrinkles forehead
NS - facial N temporal branches (CN VII)
BS - supraorbital supratrochlear branches of opthalmic artery

Occipitalis

O - Occipital bone - mastoid process (Temporalis)
I - skull aponeurosis
A - draws scalp back
NS - facial N postauricular branch
BS - facial

Erector Spinae (ES) - Iliocostalis, Longissimus, Spinalis

- see muscles of the Back - muscles are also each listed separately

Extensor Carpi Radialis Brevis

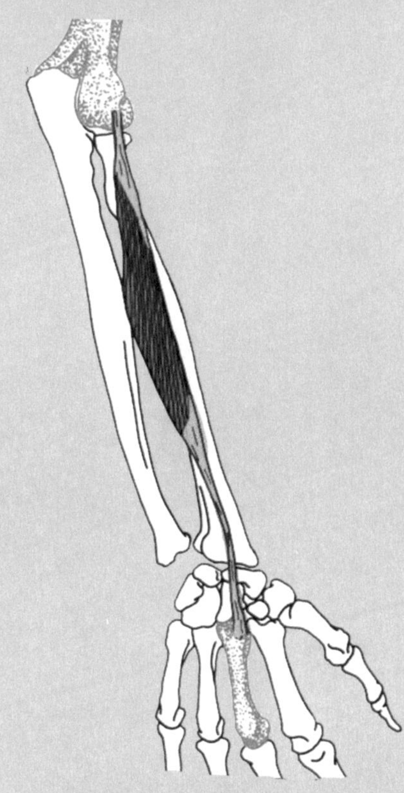

O - lateral epicondyle (Humerus)
I - dorsal base of MC 3
A - extension (wrist)
- radial deviation of hand
NS - radial N (C6-8)
BS - radial
- radial recurrent
T - lift hand from table against R
- move flat hand towards thumb against R

A
B
C
D
E
F
G
H
I
J
K
L
M
N
O
P
Q
R
S
T
U
V
W
X
Y
Z

Extensor Carpi Radialis Longus

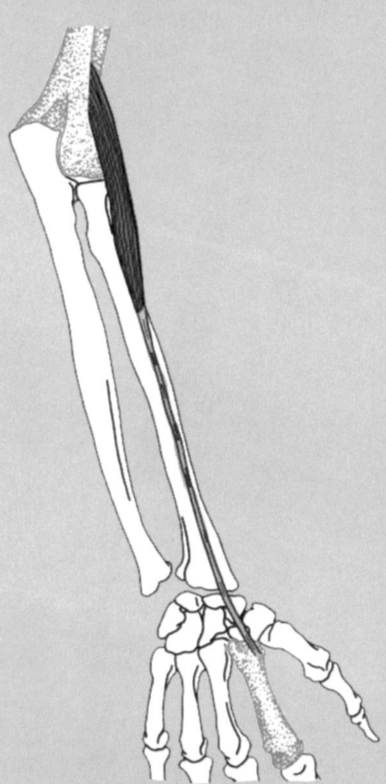

O - lateral supracondylar ridge (Humerus)
I - dorsal base of MC 2
A - extension (wrist)
NS - radial N (C6-8)
BS - radial, radial recurrent
- posterior interosseus
T - lift hand from table against R

Extensor Carpis Ulnaris

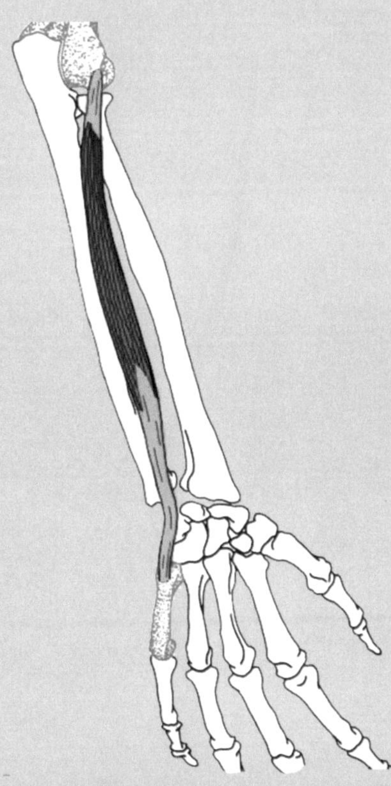

O - lateral epicondyle (Humerus)
- interosseus membrane from posterior surface

I - medial base of MC5

A - extension (wrist)
- lateral deviation of hand

NS - radial N (C6-8)

BS - ulnar

T - lift hand from table against R

Extensor Digiti Minimi

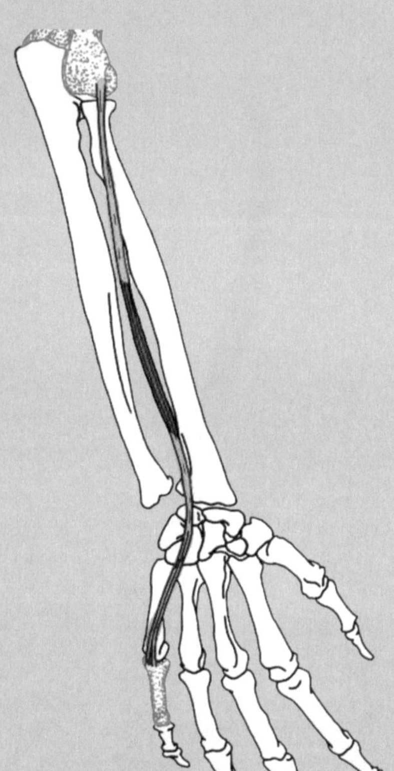

O - lateral epicondyle (Humerus)
I - dorsal Phalanx 1, Digit 5 via Extensor Digitorum tendon
A - extension (forearm, hand & Digit 5)
  - abduction (Digit 5)
NS - radial N, deep radial N (posterior interosseus N) (C7-8)
BS - ulnar
T - abduct little finger against R

Extensor Digitorum

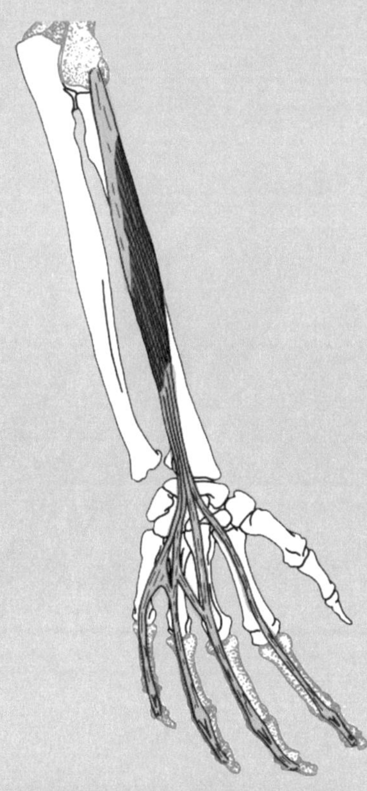

O - lateral epicondyle (Humerus)
I - 4 tendons arise and are attached to dorsal base of Phalanges 2-3 & Digits 2-5
A - extension (forearm, hand & Digits2-5)
NS - radial N, deep radial N (posterior interosseus N) (C7-8)
BS - ulnar
T - extend hand from fist against R

A
B
C
D
E
F
G
H
I
J
K
L
M
N
O
P
Q
R
S
T
U
V
W
X
Y
Z

Extensor Digitorum Brevis

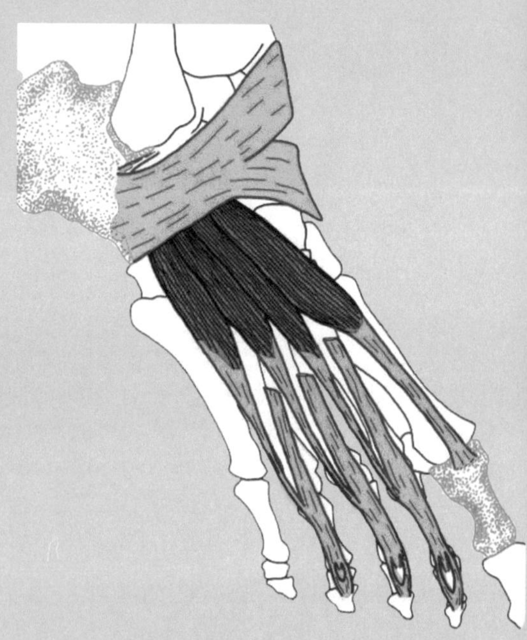

O - superio-lateral surface of Calcaneus
- inferior retinaculum

I - 4 tendons arise and are attached to dorsal base of Phalanx 1 & Digits 2-4

A - extension (Digits1-4)

NS - deep peroneal N (L5-S1)

BS - dorsalis pedis
- lateral tarsal

T - lift toes with foot on floor from upright patient

Extensor Digitorum Longus

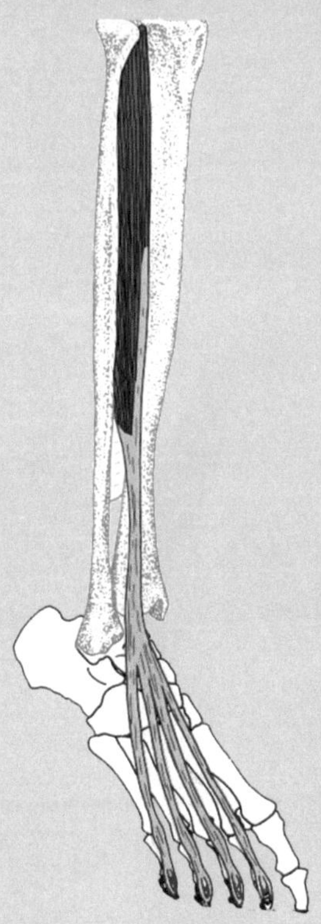

O - anterior surfaces of Tibia & Fibula
  - interosseus membrane
I - 4 tendons arise and are attached to dorsal base of Phalanges & Digits 2-5
A - extension (Digits1-4)
  - dorsiflexion of the ankle
NS - deep peroneal N, anterior tibial N (L4-S1)
BS - anterior tibial
T - lift foot and toes with heel on floor from upright patient
  - walk / stand on heels

Extensor Hallicus Brevis

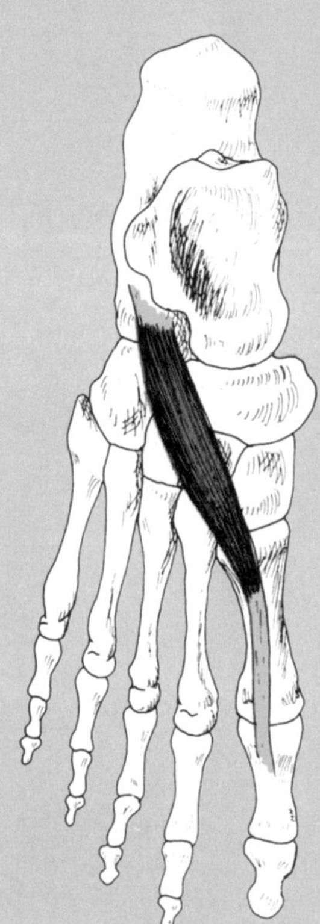

O - superio-lateral surface of Calcaneus
  - inferior retinaculum
I - dorsal base of Phalanx 1 & Digit 1
A - extension (Digit1)
NS - deep peroneal N (S1-2)
BS - dorsalis pedis
  - medial tarsal
T - uncurl big toe against R

Extensor Hallicus Longus

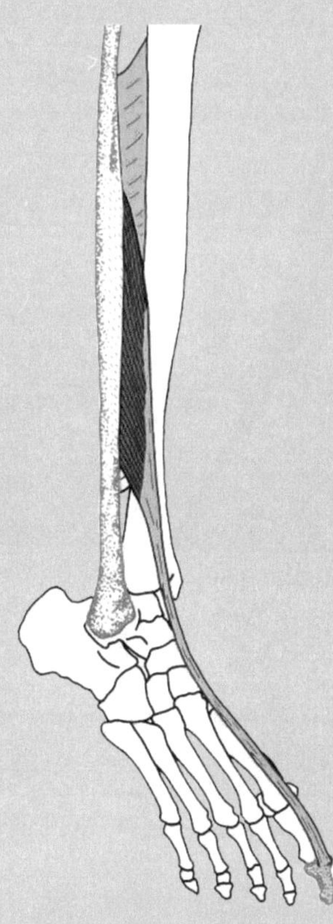

O - anterior Fibula
I - Phalanx 2 & Digit 1
A - extension (Digit 1)
 - dorsiflexion (ankle)
NS - deep peroneal N (S1-2)
BS - dorsalis pedis
 - anterior tibial
T - lift big toe from floor from upright patient
 - extend big toe

Extensor Indicis

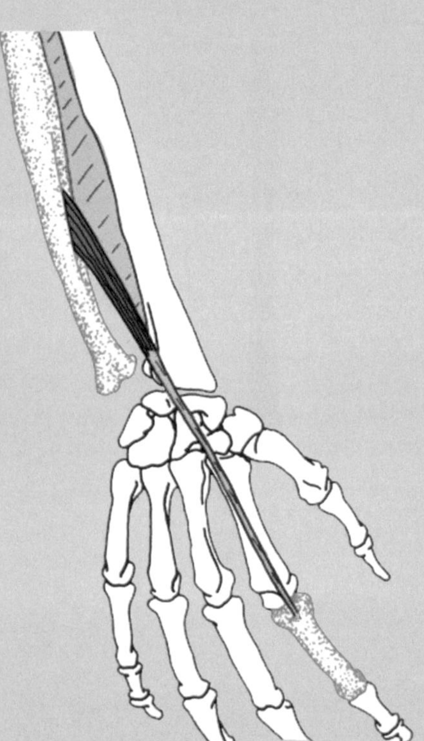

O - dorsal distal ½ of Ulna
- posterior distal surface of interosseus membrane

I - dorsal base of Phalanges 2-3 & Digit 2 via extensor digitorum tendon

A - extension (hand & Digit 2)

NS - radial N (C7-T1)

BS - ulnar

T - extend curled hand & index finger

Extensor Pollicis Brevis

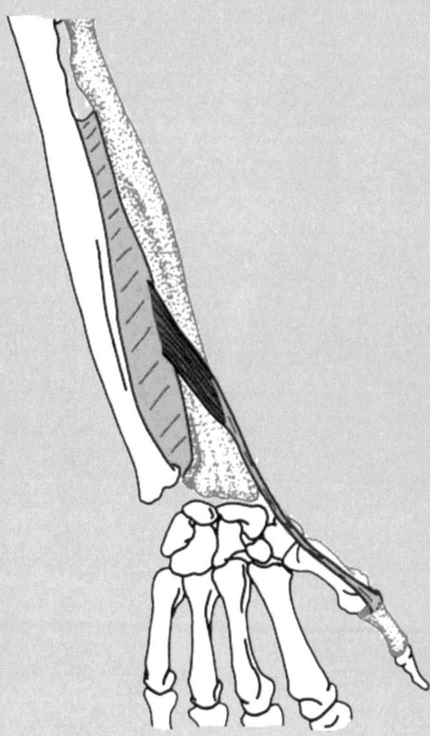

O - dorsal surface of Radius
I - dorsal base of Phalanx 1 & Digit 1
A - extension and abduction (hand & thumb)
NS - radial N, deep radial (= posterior interosseus N) (C6-7)
BS - ulnar
T - open curled thumb against R

Extensor Pollicis Longus

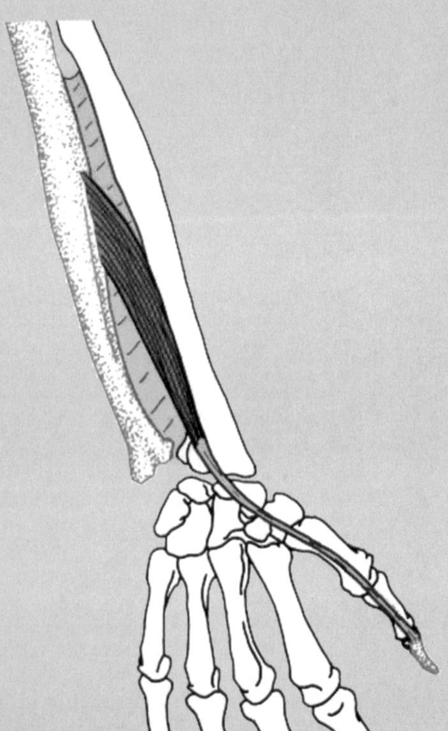

O - dorso-lateral surface in the middle 1/3 of Ulna
- interosseus membrane

I - dorsal base of Phalanx 2 & Digit 1

A - extension and abduction (hand & thumb)

NS - radial N, deep radial (= posterior interosseus N) (C6-7)

BS - ulnar

T - open curled thumb against R

External Anal Sphincter - *see Sphincter Ani*
External Intercostals - *see Intercostals*
External Obliques - *see Obliquuis Abdominus Externus*
Extrinsic Auricular Muscles - *see Auricularis*
Extrinsic Ocular muscles - *see the muscles of the Eye*

Flexor Carpi Radialis

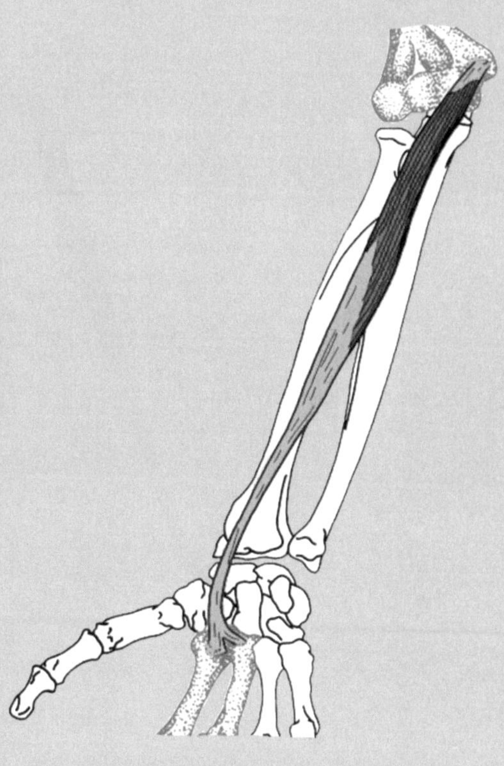

O - medial condyle (Humerus)
I - dorsal base of MC 2-3
A - flexion (forearm & hand)
NS - median N (C6-7)
BS - radial, radial recurrent
T - lift up forearm lying flat on a table against R

Flexor Carpi Ulnaris

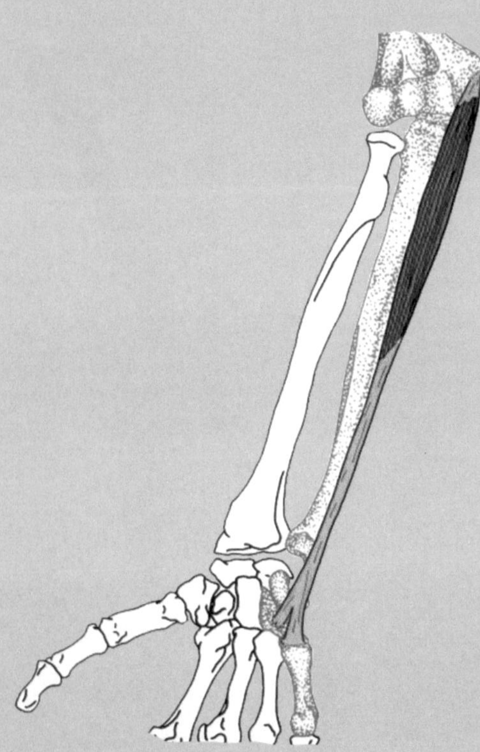

O - medial condyle (Humerus)
- proximal posterior (Ulna)

I - Pisiform
- base of MC 5

A - flexion (forearm & hand)

NS - ulnar N (C7-8)

BS - posterior ulnar recurrent

T - lift up forearm lying flat on a table against R

Flexor Digiti Minimi Brevis (foot)

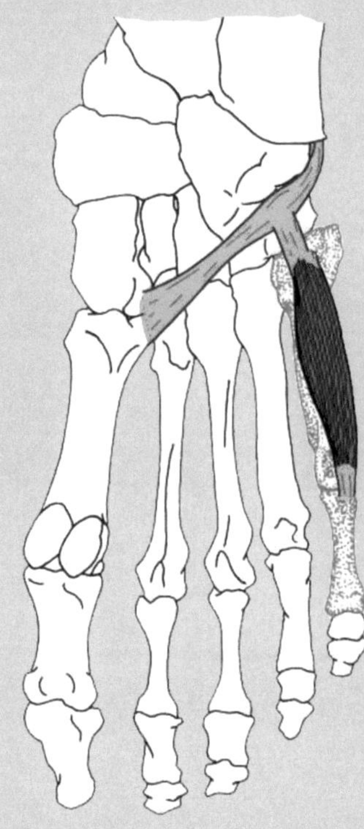

O - base MT 5, sheath of Peroneus Longus
I - base of Phalanx 1 & Digit 5
A - flexion (foot & little toe)
NS - lateral plantar N (L4-5)
BS - lateral plantar
T - curl up little toe

A
B
C
D
E
F
G
H
I
J
K
L
M
N
O
P
Q
R
S
T
U
V
W
X
Y
Z

Flexor Digiti Minimi Brevis (hand)

Hypothenar eminence

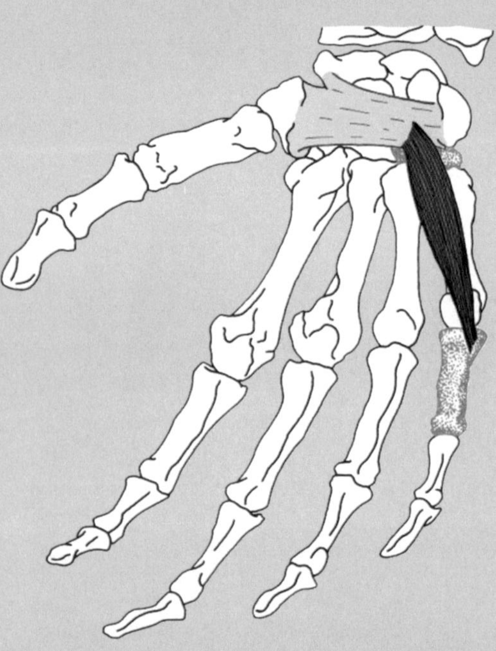

O - flexor retinaculum
  - Hamulus & Hamate
I - ulnar side of Phalanx 1, Digit 5
A - flexion of little finger
NS - ulnar N, (C8-T1)
BS - ulnar
T - flex little finger against R

Flexor Digitorum Brevis (foot)

first layer of the sole of the foot

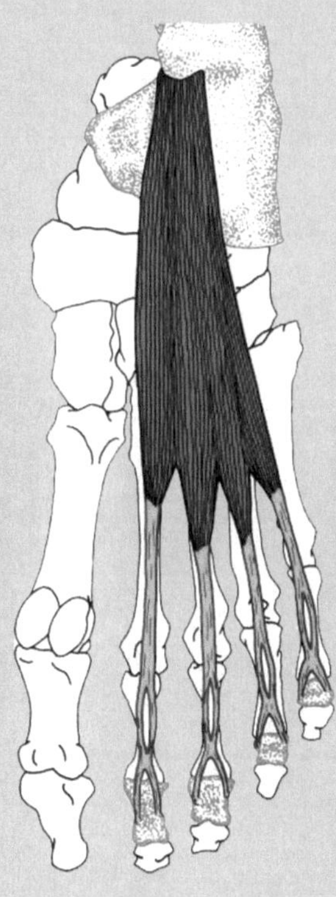

O - tuberosity of the Calcaneus
I - sides of the middle phalanx of digits 2-4 ±5
A - flexion of the foot and toes
NS - medial plantar N (L4-5)
BS - medial and lateral plantar
T - curl toes

Flexor Digitorum Longus (foot)

second layer of the muscles of the sole of the foot

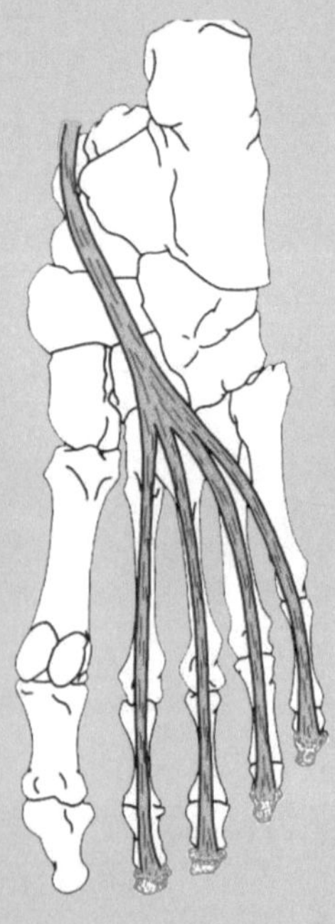

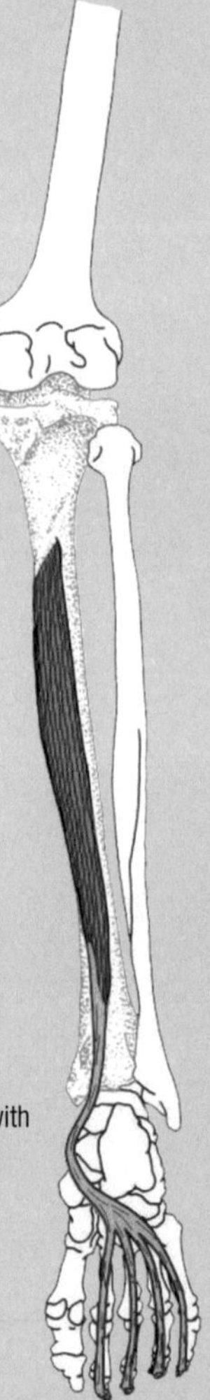

O - posterior Tibia
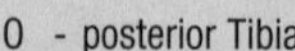
I - base of Phalanx 3 & Digits 2-5
A - flexion & plantar flexion of the foot
NS - posterior tibial N (S2-3)
BS - posterior tibial
T - push toes into hand on the prone patient with feet over the end. ie plantar flex against R

Flexor Digitorum Profundus (hand)

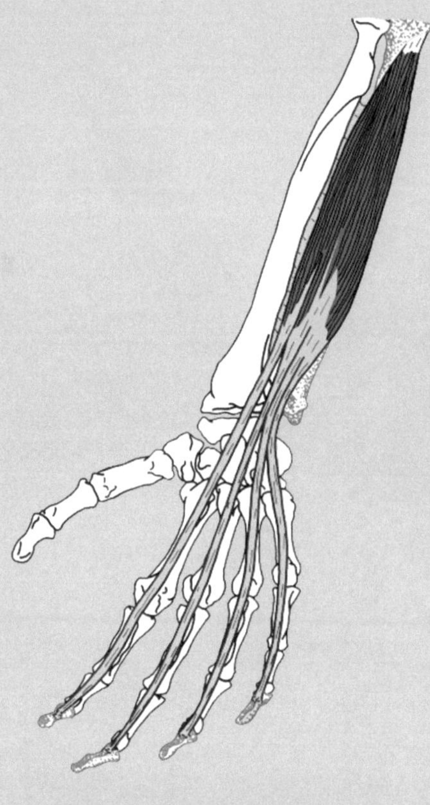

O - proximal 2/3 on anterior surface of Ulna
  - coronoid process (Ulna)
I - ulnar side of Phalanx 3, Digits 2-5
A - flexion of hand & fingers 2-5
NS - median & ulnar Ns, (C8-T1)
BS - ulnar
T - flex fingers against R

Flexor Digitorum Superficialis (hand)

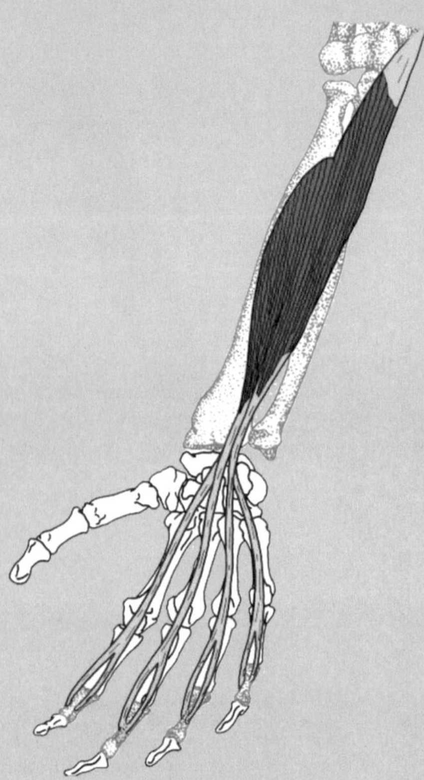

O - medial epicondyle (Humerus)
- anterior onlique line (Radius)
- coronoid process (Ulna)

I - Phalanx 2, Digits 2-5

A - flexion (forearm, hand and fingers 2-5)

NS - median N, (C7-8)

BS - ulnar, radial

T - flex fingers against R

Flexor Hallucis Brevis (foot)
third layer of the sole of the foot

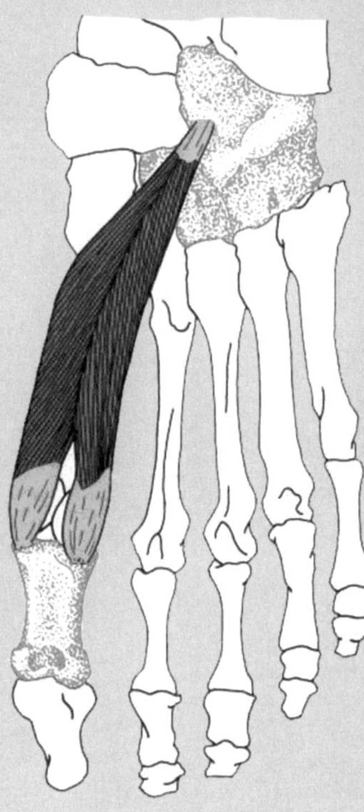

O - plantar surface of the Cuboid
- lateral Cuniform
- Tibialis Posterior tendon

I - both sides of Phalanx 1 & Digit 1
A - flexion (big toe)
NS - 1st plantar digital N (L4-S3)
BS - medial plantar
T - curl up big toe

A
B
C
D
E
F
G
H
I
J
K
L
M
N
O
P
Q
R
S
T
U
V
W
X
Y
Z

Flexor Hallucis Longus (foot)
second layer of the sole of the foot

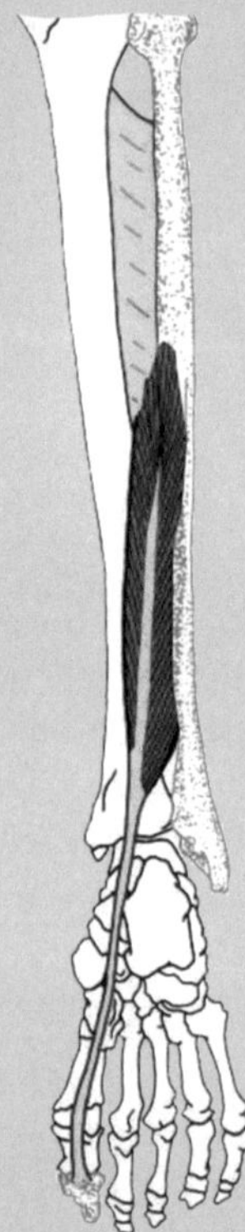

O - lower posterior Fibula
I - base of Phalanx 2 & Digit 1
A - flexion & plantarflexion of the foot
- inversion of the foot
- medial stabilization of the ankle
- support for longitudinal ligament of arch
NS - posterior tibial N (S2-3)
BS - posterior tibial
- peroneal
T - plantarflex foot against R
- flex big toe against R

Flexor Pollicis Brevis

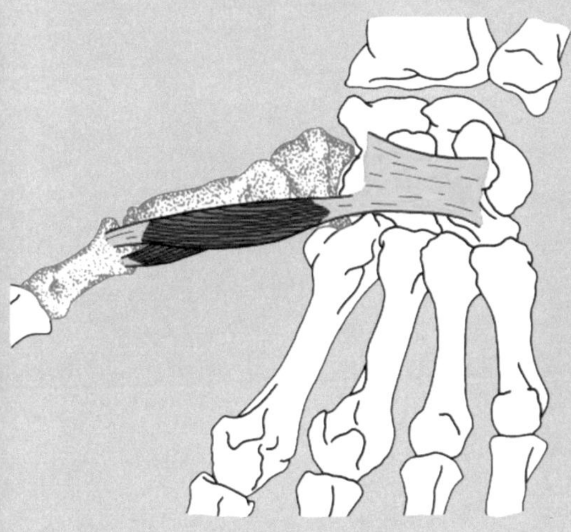

O - flexor retinaculum
  - Trapezium ridge
I - lateral base of Phalanx 1, Digit 1
A - flexion of thumb
NS - median & ulnar Ns (C6-T1)
BS - radial - palmar digital branches
T - flex thumb against R

Flexor Pollicis Longus

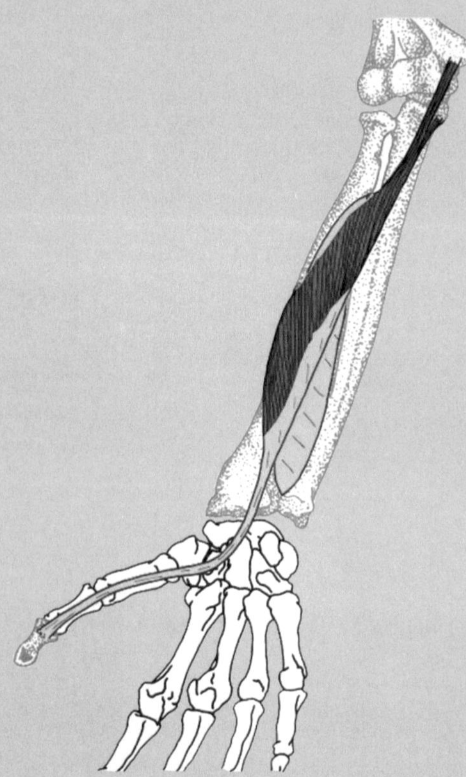

O - anterior surface of middle 1/2 of Radius
- interosseus membrane (b/n Radius & Ulna)
- coronoid process (Ulna)

I - Phalanx 2, Digit 1

A - flexion (hand & thumb)

NS - median N, (C8-T1)

BS - ulnar

T - flex hand and thumb against R

Frontalis - ***see Epicranius***

Gastrocnemius

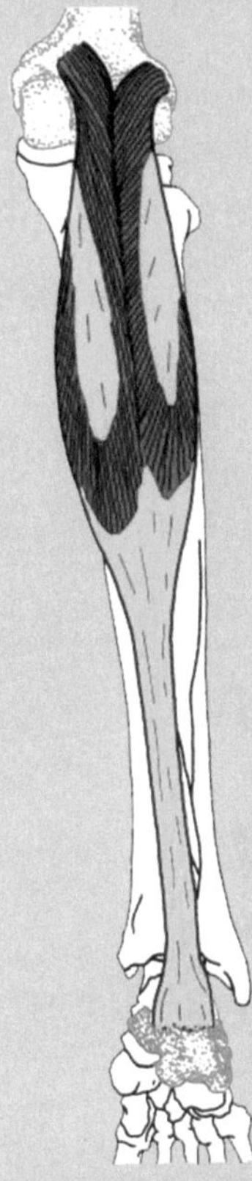

O - posterior condyles (Femur) via 2 heads
medial & lateral

I - Archille's tendon to tuberosity of Calcaneus

A - knee flexion
- plantar flexion and inversion of the foot

NS - tibial N (S1-2)

BS - popliteal

T - flex knee against R

Gemellus

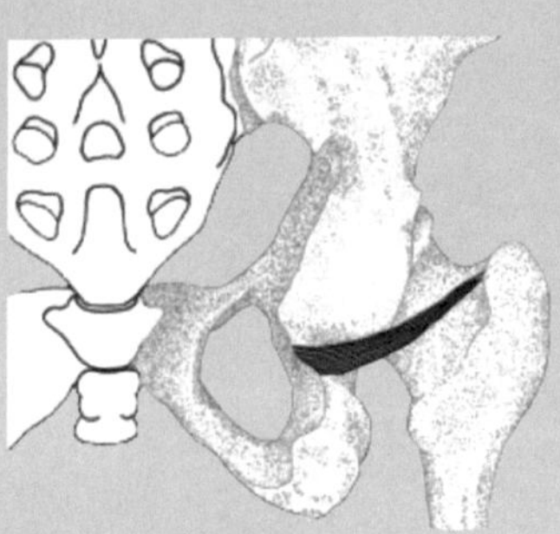

Inferior

O - ischeal tuberosity (hip)
I - medial surface of the greater trochanter (Femur)
A - lateral rotation
NS - N to Quadratus Femoris branch of (L4-S1)
BS - inferior gluteal
T - rotate hip against R

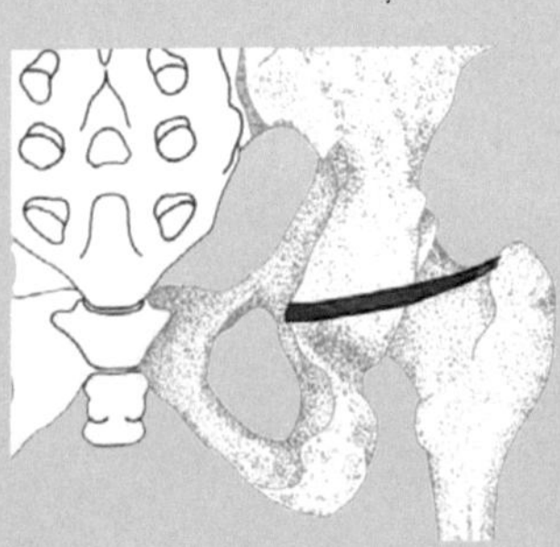

Superior

O - ischeal spine (hip)
I - medial surface of the greater trochanter (Femur)
A - lateral rotation
NS - N to Obturator Internus, SP (L4-S1)
BS - inferior gluteal
T - rotate hip against R

Genioglossus - *see Tongue Muscles*
Geniohyoid - *see Thyro / Hyoid Muscles*

Gluteus Maximus

A B C D E F **G** H I J K L M N O P Q R S T U V W X Y Z

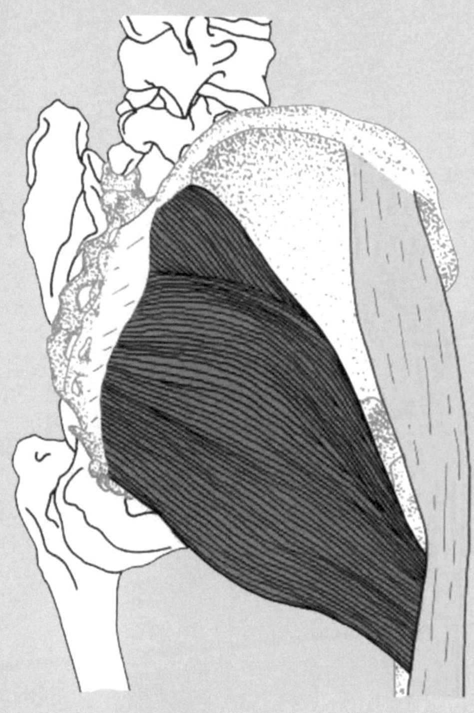

O - posterior crest of the Ileum (hip)
  - Sacrum & Coccyx
I - greater trochanter (Femur)
  - Tensor Fascia Lata
  - linea aspera (Femur)
A - lateral rotation (hip)
  - extension (thigh)
NS - inferior gluteal N (L5-S2)
  - angiococcygeal Ns dorsal sacral Ns (S1-5)
BS - superior gluteal
T - extend leg against R or in the standing patient

Gluteus Medius

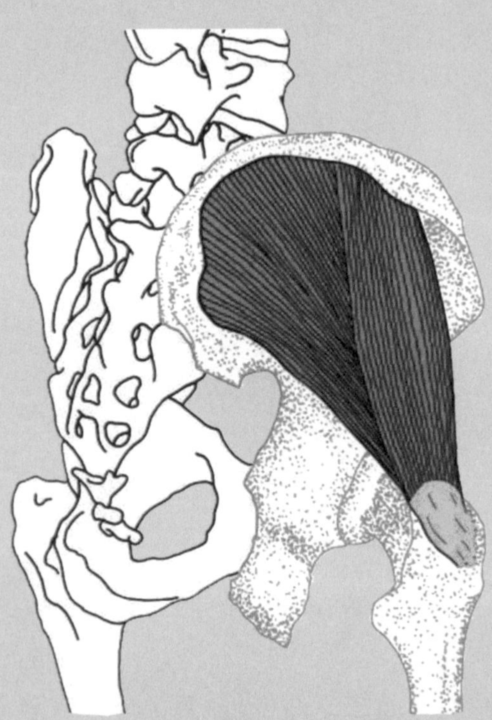

O - posterior crest of the Ileum b/n upper 2 gluteal lines (hip)
I - lateral surface of the greater trochanter (Femur)
A - abduction (Femur)
  - medial rotator (hip)
NS - superior gluteal N (L5-S1)
BS - superior gluteal
T - extend leg against R or in the standing patient

Gluteus Minimus

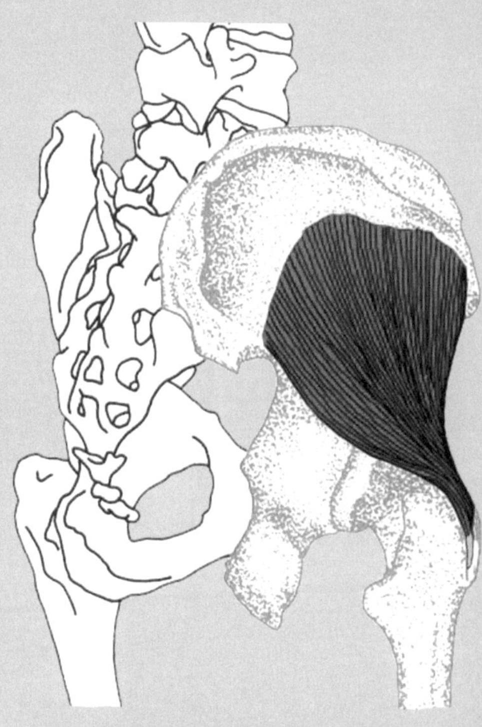

O - posterior crest of the Ileum b/n upper 2 gluteal lines (hip)
  - margin of sciatic notch
I - anterolateral border of the greater trochanter (Femur)
A - abduction (hip)
  - pelvic stabilizer
NS - superior gluteal N (L5-S1)
BS - superior gluteal
T - extend leg against R or in the standing patient
  - test balance on one leg

Gracillis

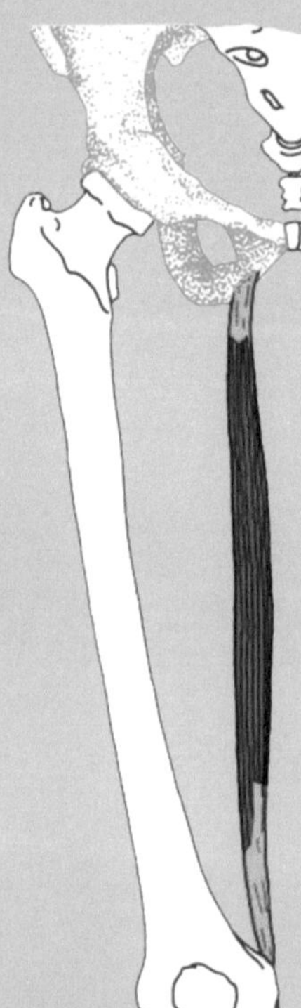

O - pubic symphysis (hip)
I - anteromedial surface of the Tibia
A - flexion (hip)
- adduction (hip)
NS - obturator N (L2-4)
BS - deep femoral
- obturator
- medial femoral circumflex
T - flex hip against R

Hyoid muscles - Geniohyoid, Mylohyoid, Omohyoid, Sternohyoid
- see individual listings and the Thyro /Hyoid muscles
Hypoglossus - *see Tongue Muscles*

Iliacus
part of Iliopsoas

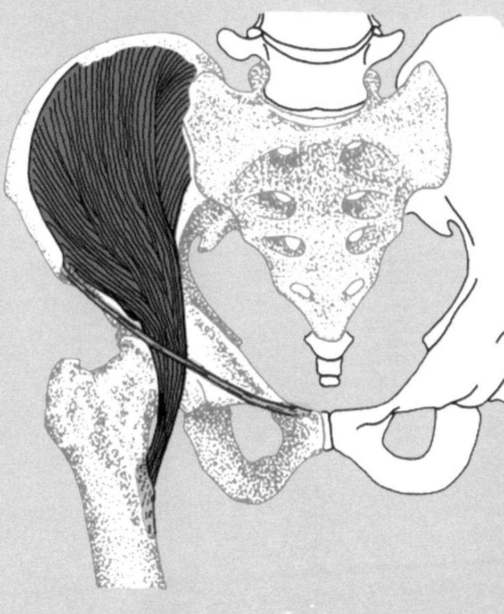

O - iliac fossa (hip)
I - lesser trochanter (Femur)
A - flexion (hip) from supine position
  - anterior pelvic tilt (hip)
NS - femoral N (L2-3)
BS - deep femoral
  - obturator
  - medial femoral circumflex
T - flex hip in the supine patient

Iliocostalis
part of the ES

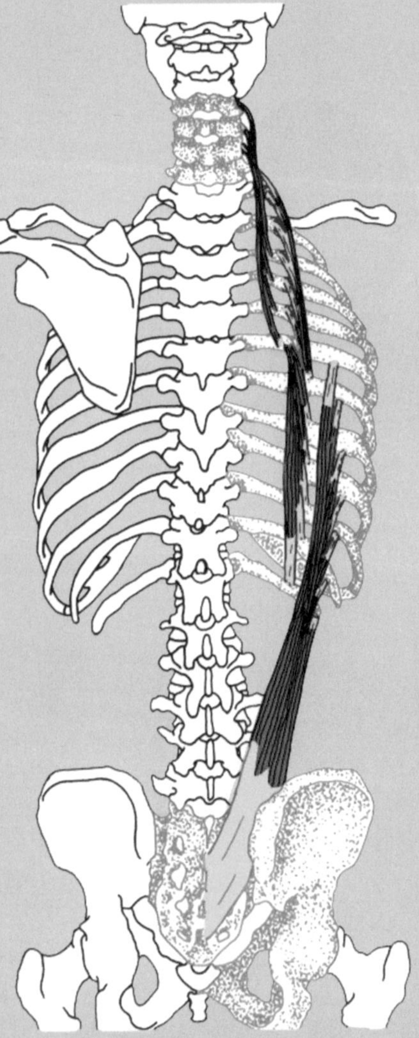

Iliocostalis

Cervicis

O - angles of ribs 3-6
I - TPs of cervical VBs 4-6
A - bilateral action - extension of cervical VC
- unilateral action - lateral flexion of cervical VC
NS - segmental doral branches of SNs
BS - segmental dorsal branches of the carotids
T - extend neck against R and laterally flex against R

Thoracis

O - angles of ribs 6-12
I - TP of cervical VB C7
- angles of ribs 1-6
A - bilateral action - forceful contraction of the ribs for inspiration
- unilateral action - lat. flexion of VC (largely stopped by the ribs)
NS - segmental dorsal branches of SNs
BS - segmental dorsal branches of descending aorta
T - ask patient to inspire forcefully

Lumborum

O - sacral crest and medial parts of the iliac crests
I - angles of ribs 3-6 lateral to Thoracis
A - bilateral forced inspiration, extension of the VC
- unilateral lateral flexion of the VC
NS - segmental dorsal branches of SNs
BS - segmental dorsal branches of descending aorta, iliacs, lumbar and sacral vessels

Iliopsoas = Iliacus + Psoas - *see Iliacus and Psoas*
Iliotibial Tract - *see Tensor Fascia Lata*
Incisivus Labii - Inferior, Superior - *see the muscles of the Face*
Inferior Lingualis - *see the muscles of the Tongue*
Inferior Oblique - *see the muscles of the Eye*
Inferior Pharyngeal Constrictor - *see Pharyngeal Constrictors*
Inferior rectus - *see the muscles of the Eye*

A B C D E F G H **I** J K L M N O P Q R S T U V W X Y Z

Infraspinatus

part of the shoulder girdle - rotator cuff muscles

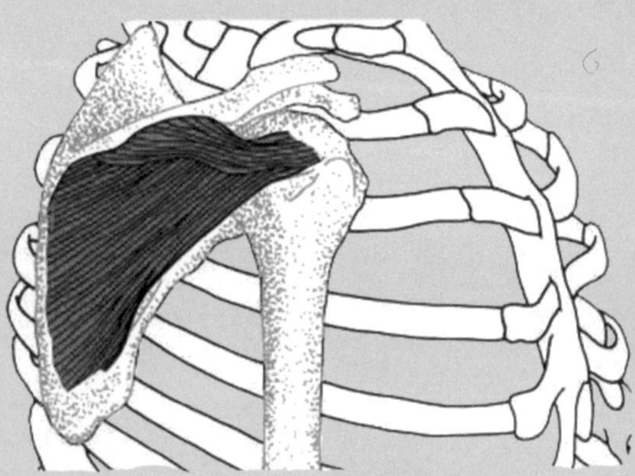

O - medial 2/3 of infraspinous fossa (Scapula)
I - greater tuberosity (Humerus)
A - lateral rotation
- horizontal abduction (shoulder)
NS - suprascapular N (C4-6)
BS - suprascapular
- transverse cervical
- scapular cirumflex
T - with anterior horizontal arm move around against R

Innermost Intercostals - *see Intercostals*
Internal intercostals - *see Intercostals*
Internal Obliques - *see Obliquuis Abdominus Internus*

Intercostals

as a group the muscles b/n ribs

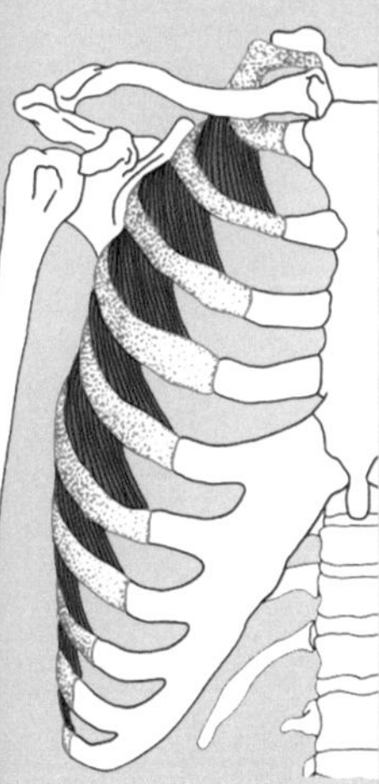

External

O - costal groove of the rib
I - superior surface of the rib below
A - draws adjacent ribs up and closer together
- increases thoracic volume with contracted Diaphragm

NS - segmental - anterior branches of SNs (T1-12)
BS - internal thoracic
- intercostal branches

T - movement of rib cage with breathing

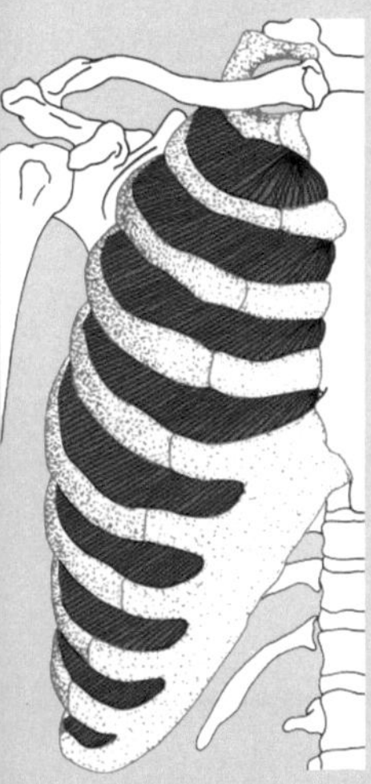

Internal

O - inferior border of the rib
I - superior surface of the rib below
A - draws adjacent ribs down and closer together
- decreases thoracic volume with relaxed Diaphragm
- flexion of the thorax

NS - segmental - anterior branches of SNs (T1-12)
BS - internal thoracic
- intercostal branches

T - movement of rib cage with breathing

Intimi = Innermost Intercostals - see *Intercostals*

Interspinalis
cervical, thoracic and lumbar

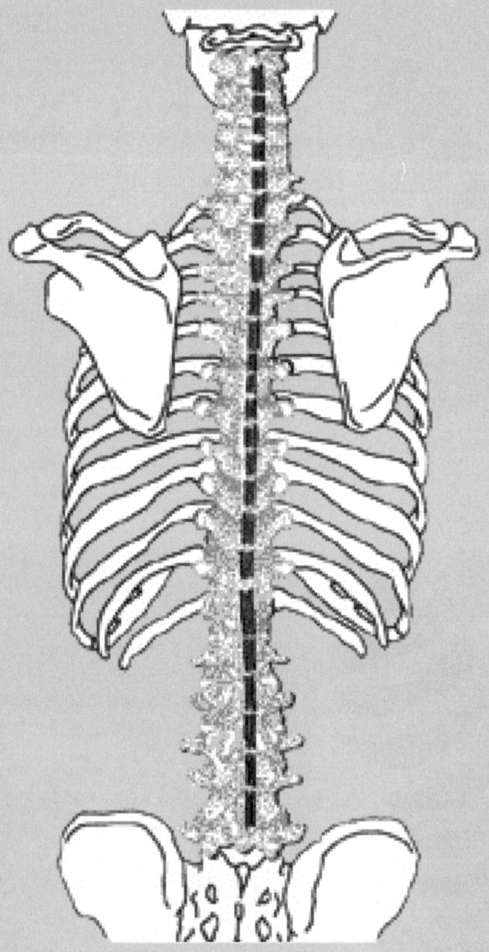

O - cervical SP of C3-7
- thoracic SP of T2-12
- lumbar SP L2-5

I - SP of the immediate VB above

A - draws adjacent VBs together extending the VC

NS - segmental - dorsal branches of relative SNs (C1-L5)

BS - cervical - branches of the internal carotid
- thoracic - dorsal branches of the decending aorta
- lumbar - dorsal branches of the iliacs

Interossei - Muscles groups - Dorsal, Palmer (hand), Dorsal, Plantar (foot) - *see individual listings of these muscles*
O & I listed individually - as a group these muscles lie b/n the MT or the MC bones of the hands or feet.
A listed individually - as a group they assist in abduction (dorsal) / adduction (plantar, palmar) of the toes /fingers of the foot or hand.
NS the digital branches of the Ns supplying the hand or foot
BS the digital branches of the BVs supplying the hand or foot coming from arches in the hand or foot

Intertranversarii

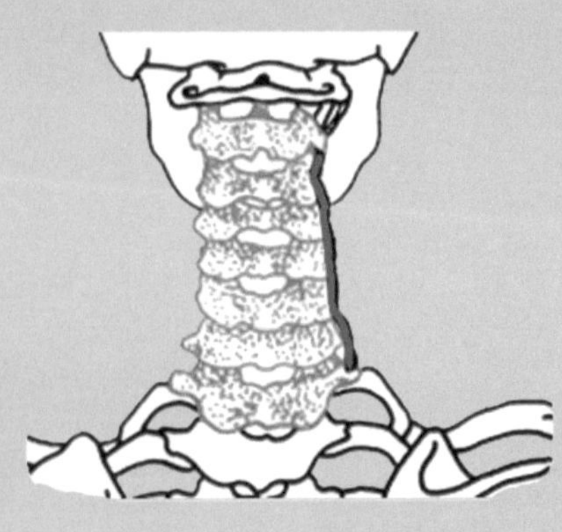

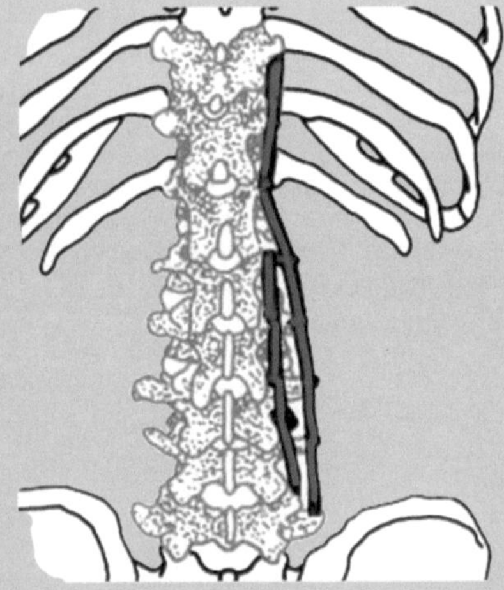

O - cervical - TP of C1-T1 on the anterior & posterior surfaces
- thoracic - TP of T11- L1 on the posterior surface only
- lumbar - TP on the lateral surface and mamillary bodies of L1-5
I - TP of the immediate VB above on the same surface
A - draws adjacent VBs together extending the VC
NS - segmental - ventral branches of relative SNs
BS - cervical - branches of the internal carotid
- thoracic - dorsal branches of the decending aorta
- lumbar - dorsal branches of the iliacs

Intrinsic Auricular Muscles - Stapedius
Intrinsic Ocular Muscles - Ciliarus, Recti, Sphincter Pupillae - *see the muscles of the Eye*
Ischiocavernosus - *see the muscles of the Perineum*
Lateral Cricoarytenoid - *see the muscles of the Larynx*

Latissimus Dorsi

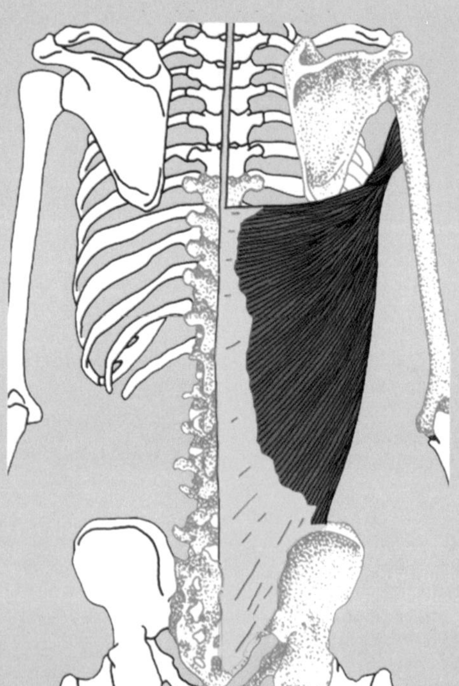

O - spines of T7-L5
- sacrum
- iliac crest
- ribs 10-12

I - floor of the bicipital groove (Humerus)

A - extension (arm)
- adduction and horizontal abduction (arm)

NS - thoracodorsal N (C6-8)

BS - transverse cervical
- subscapluar

T - extend arm against R

Levator Ani - *see the muscles of the Pelvis and Perineum*
Levator Anguli Oris - *see the muscles of the Face*
Levator Palpabrae Superioris - *see the muscles of the Eye*

Levator Costi
Brevis

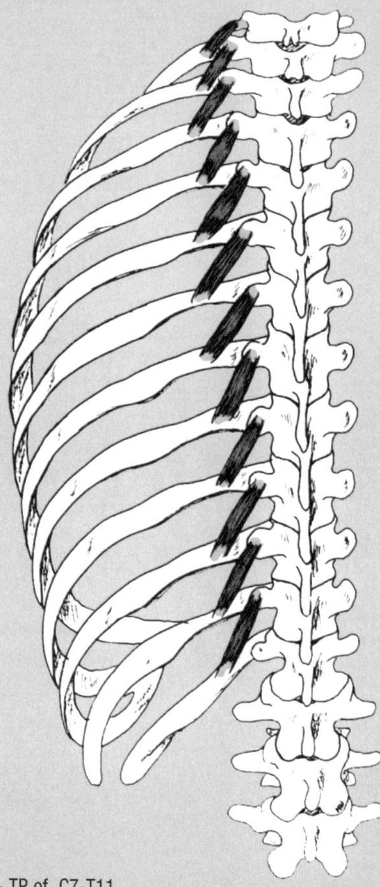

O - TP of C7-T11

I - outer surface of the rib immediately inferior b/n tubercle and angle

A - elevate ribs in inspiration
- extend and laterally flex VC in thoracic region

NS - segmental dorsal branches of the corresponding SNs (C7-T11)

BS - segmental dorsal branches of the descending aorta

Levator Costi

Longus

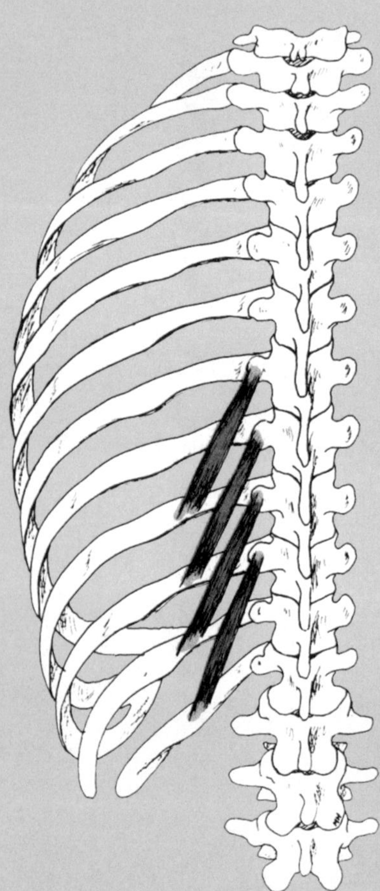

O - TP of T7-T10

I - outer surface of the ribs 2-3 below b/n tubercle and angle

A - elevate ribs in inspiration
- extend and laterally flex VC in thoracic region
- rotation of the VC

NS - segmental dorsal branches of the corresponding SNs (T7-T11)

BS - segmental dorsal branches of the descending aorta

Levator Scapulae

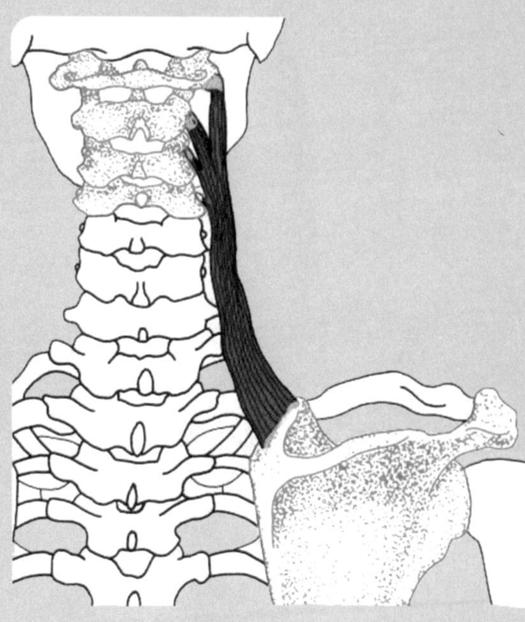

O - TP of C1-4 (5)
I - medial border of Scapula to the spine
A - elevate (shoulders) unilateral or bilateral
  - lateral flexion, medial rotation (neck) unilateral
NS - dorsal scapular N (C5)
  - dorsal branches of the SNs (C3-4)
  - N to Levator Scapulae
BS - segmental dorsal branches of the descending aorta

Levator Veli Palatini - *see the Soft Palate Muscles*
Lingualis - Inferior, Transverse & Vertical - *see the Tongue Muscles*

Longissimus

Capitus, Cerivcis & Thoracis - part of ES

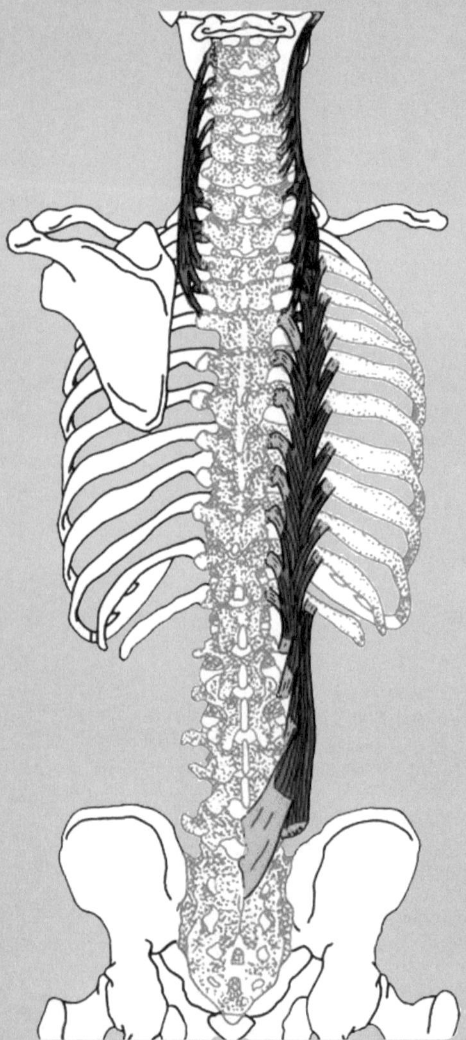

O - Capitus - TP of C1-5
Cervicis -TP of C1-5
Thoracis - TP of T1-5
I - Capitus - mastoid process (Temporalis)
Cervicis - TP of C2-6
Thoracis - TP of T1-12
A - extension and rotation of the VC
NS - segmental spinal roots generally the dorsal branches (C1-L5)
BS - segmental dorsal branches of the ascending cervical BVs, descending aorta and lumbar arteries
T - to stand up from touching toes w/o help
- from upright position bend to one side and the other w/o help

Longus Capitus

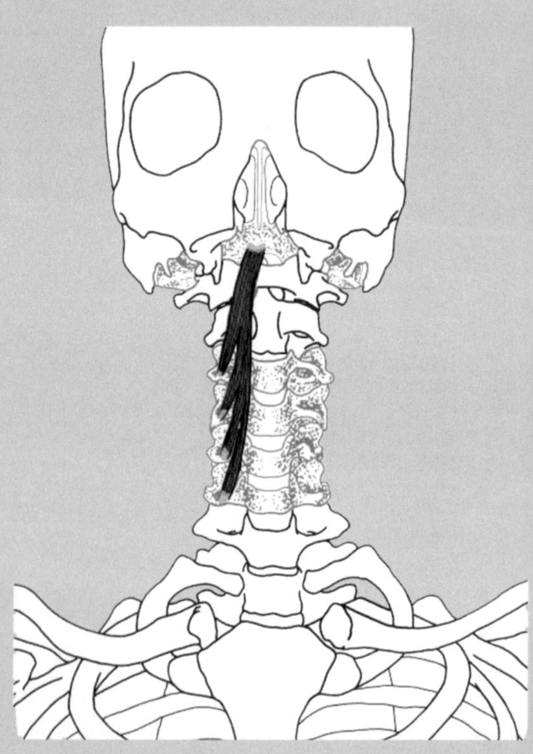

O - TP of C3-7
I - anterior surface of Occiput
A - flexion neck (bilaterally action)
  - rotation of neck (unilateral action)
NS - N to Longus Capitus (C1-C3)
BS - vertebral - maybe damaged in Whiplash accidents
T - flexion of Neck against R
  - rotation of neck against R

Longus Colli

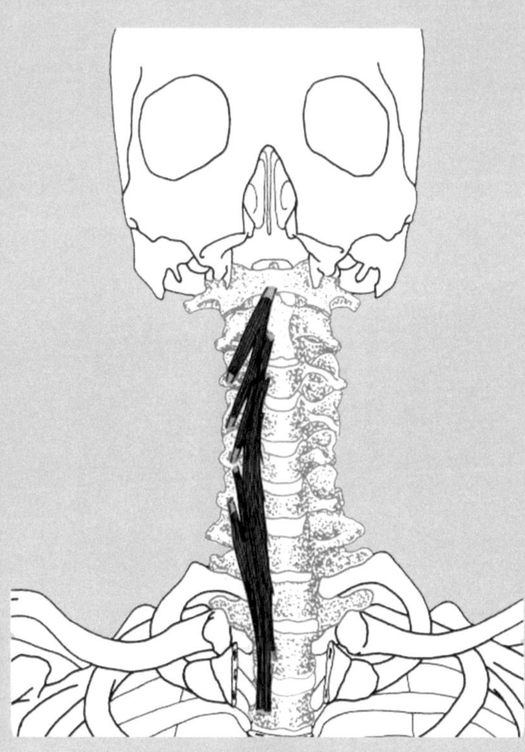

O - TP and anterior surface of C1-T3
I - anterior arch of Atlas (C1)
A - flexion neck (bilaterally action)
  - rotation of neck (unilateral action)
NS - N to Longus Colli (C1-C3)
BS - vertebral - maybe damaged in Whiplash accidents
T - flexion of Neck against R
  - rotation of neck against R

A
B
C
D
E
F
G
H
I
J
K
L
M
N
O
P
Q
R
S
T
U
V
W
X
Y
Z

Lumbricals (foot)
second layer of the soul of the foot

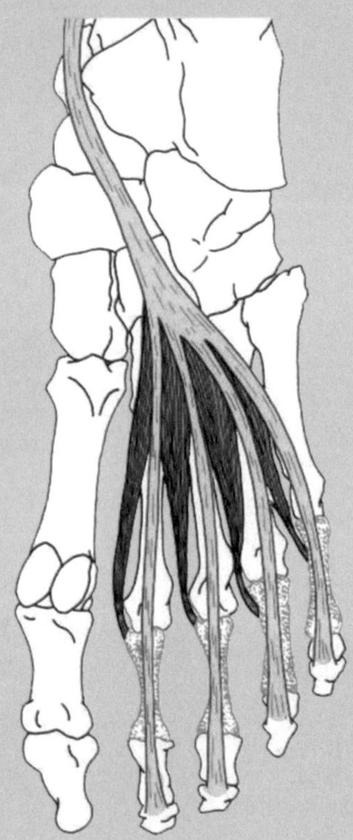

O - tendon of Flexor Digitorum Longus
I - dorsal surface of proximal Phalanges
A - flexion of toes (not big toe)
NS - medial plantar N (L4-5)
- deep lateral plantar N (S1-2)
BS - plantar metatarsal
T - to curl up toes

Lumbricals (hand)

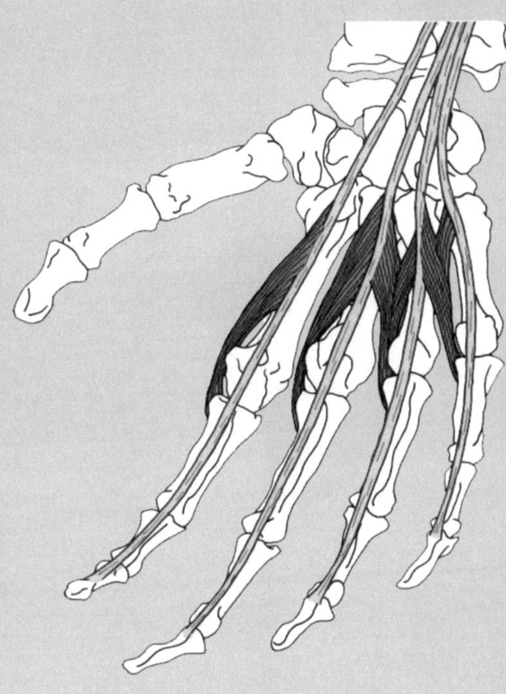

O - tendon of Flexor Digitorum Profundus to the palm
I - lateral surface of Phalanx 1 Digits 2-5
  - Extensor Digitorum tendons
A - flexion of fingers (not thumb)
NS - median & ulnar Ns (C8-T1)
BS - palmar arches deep and superficial
T - to curl up fingers

A B C D E F G H I J K L **M** N O P Q R S T U V W X Y Z

Masseter
part of the muscles of mastication

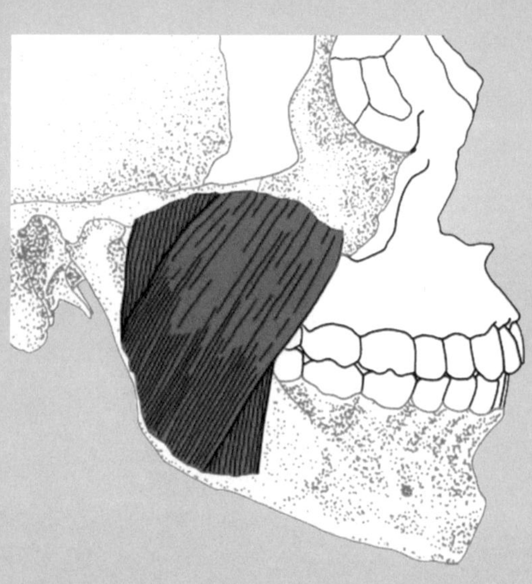

O - zygomatic arch (Maxilla)
I - Mandible
A - closes jaw
- clenches teeth
- protraction and retraction of jaw
NS - trigeminal N - mandibular branch (CN V)
BS - maxillary, facial, transverse facial
T - to clench teeth and move jaw in and out

Mentalis

part of the muscles of facial expression

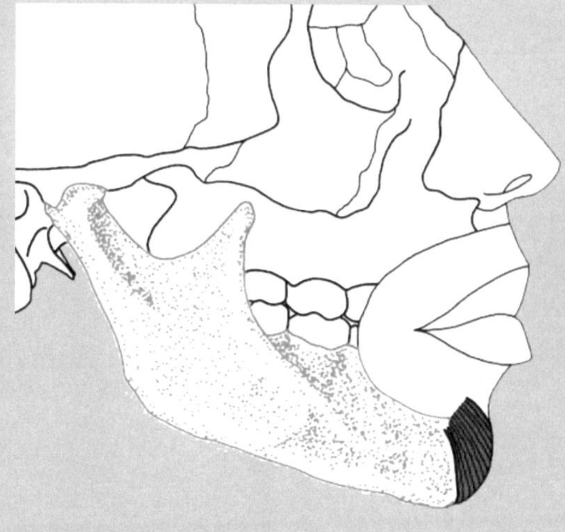

O - Mandible
I - deep fascia of the skin of the chin
A - protrudes lips
  - raises bottom lip
NS - facial N - mandibular branch (CN VII)
BS - facial - mandibular branch
T - to lift up bottom lip

Multifidus Capitus, Cervicis & Thoracis

part of deep spinal muscle layer

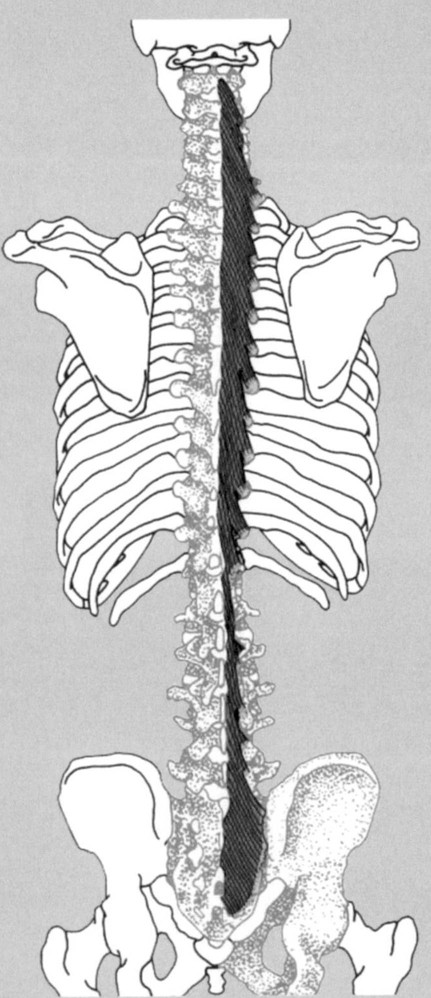

O - Capitus articular processes (zygoapophyseal) of C1-7
- Cervicis TP and intertranverse ligament T1-12
- Thoracis TP and mamillary bodies of L1-5
- posterior foraminae of Sacrum

I - SP of 2-3 VB above

A - extension and rotation of the VC
- stability of the VC

NS - segmental spinal roots generally the dorsal branches (C1-L5)

BS - segmental dorsal branches of the ascending cervical BVs, descending aorta and lumbar arteries

T - to stand up from touching toes w/o help
- from upright position bend to one side and the other w/o help

Muscularis Uvulae - *see Soft Palate Muscles*
Mylohyoid - *see Thyro / Hyoid Muscles*
Nasalis - *see the muscles of the Face*
Oblique muscles of the eye - superior / inferior - *see the muscles of the Eye*

Obliquus Abdominus - Externus

External Oblique

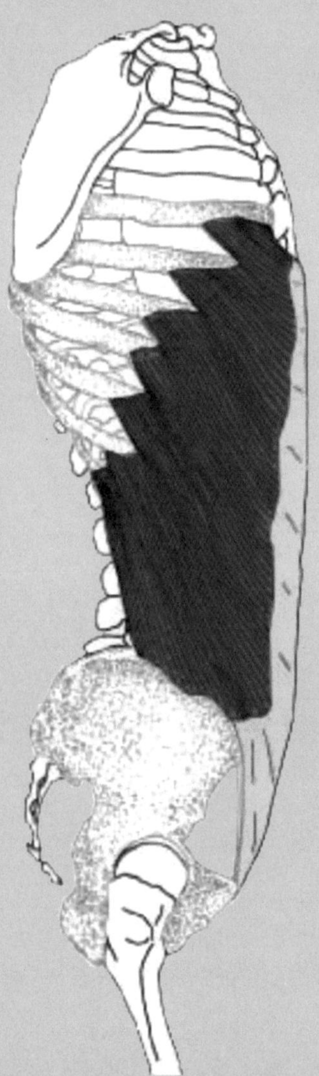

External (outer layer of abdominal muscles)

O - ribs 2 - 12 - interdigitates with Serratus Anterior
I - abdominal aponeurosis to linea alba (direction hands in front pockets)
- iliac crest (hip)
- inguinal ligament
A - **bilateral** flexion of VC
forced expiration, coughing
compression of abdominal contents
assistance in defaecation
assisting the lumbar muscles for stability of the VC
- **unilateral** rotation to opposite side
NS - segmental T8-12
- iliohypogatric, ilioinguinal Ns
BS - segmental intercostals
- ilioinguinal, iliohypogastric
T - to suck in stomach / abdomen

Obliquus Abdominis - Internus

Internal Oblique

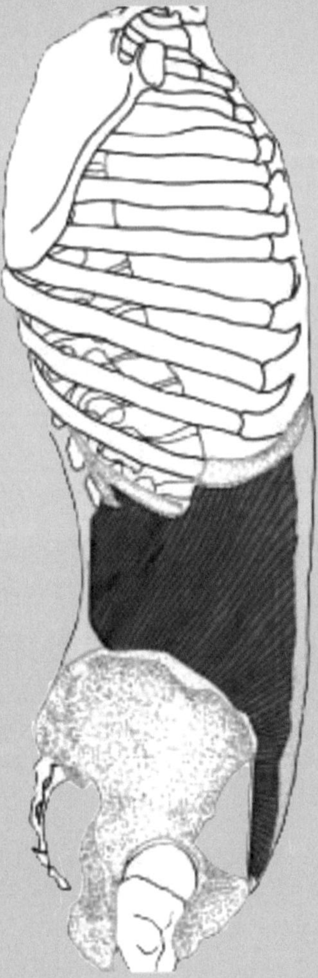

Internal (middle layer of abdominal muscles)

O - Iliac crest (hip)
  - inguinal ligament, lumbar fascia
I - abdominal aponeurosis (direction hands in back pockets)
  - lower ribs (8-12)
A - **bilateral** flexion of VC
  forced expiration, coughing
  compression of abdominal contents
  assistance in defaecation
  assisting the lumbar muscles for
  stability of the VC
  - **unilateral** rotation to opposite side
NS - segmental T8-12
  - iliohypogatric, ilioinguinal Ns
BS - segmental intercostals
  - ilioinguinal, iliohypogastric
T - to suck in stomach /abdomen

Oblquuis Capitis

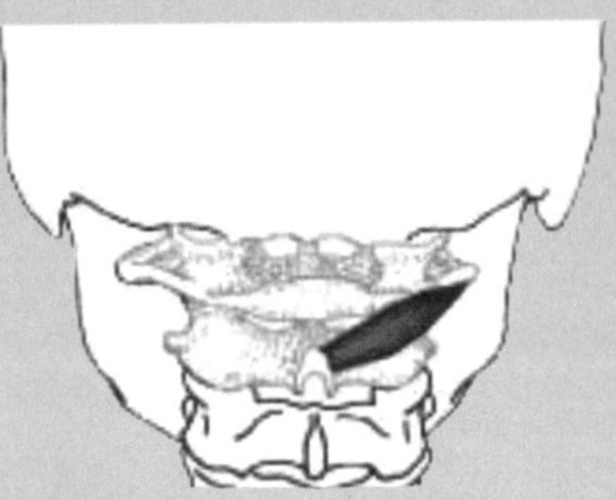

Inferior

0 - SP of C2 Axis
I - TP of C1 Atlas
A - rotates head
NS - suboccipital N (C2) and dorsal rami of C1-2
BS - vertebral

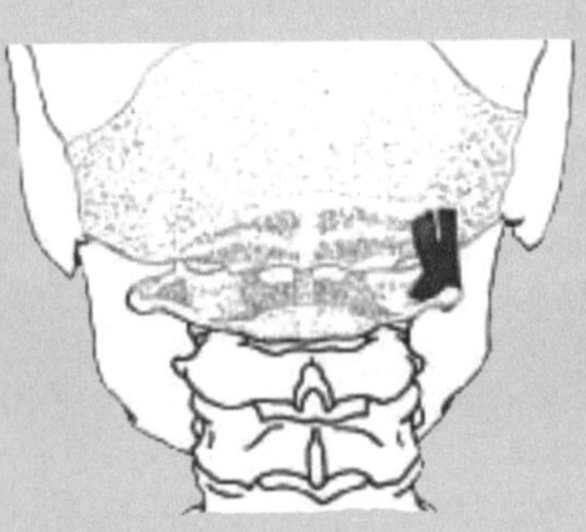

Superior

0 - TP of C1 Atlas
I - base of skull (Occiput)
A - extends head
- lateral flexion of head
NS - suboccipital N (C2) and dorsal rami of C1-2
BS - ascending cervical

T - test movements of the head ± R

Obturator Externus

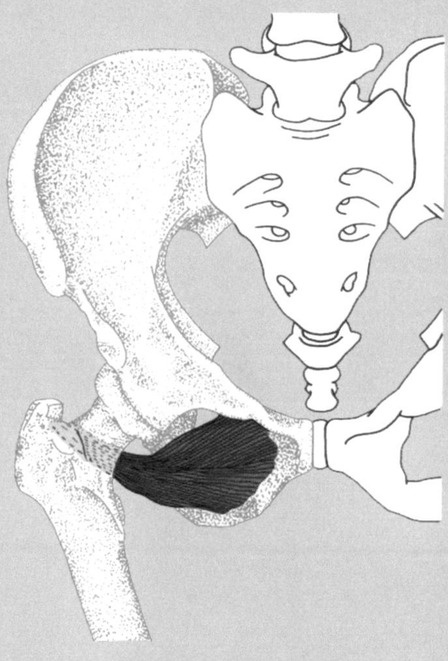

O - inferior pubic ramus and ischeal ramus (hip)
  - obturator membrane
I - trochanteric fossa (Femur)
A - lateral rotation
NS - obturator N (L3-4)
BS - obturator
  - medial femoral circumflex

Obturator Internus

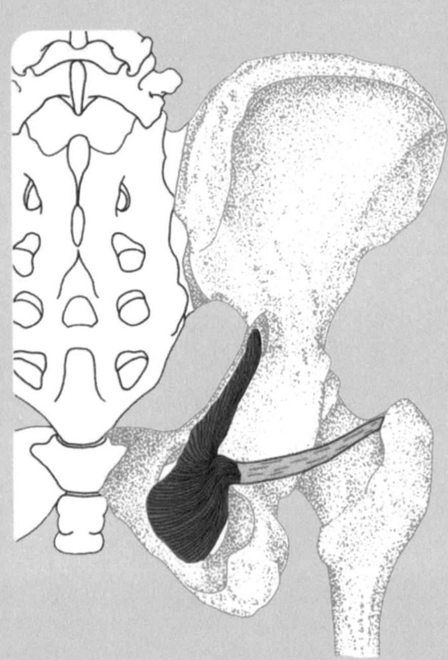

O - internal pelvic surface
  - obturator membrane through sciatic notch
I - anterior surface of medial greater trochanter (Femur)
A - lateral rotation (hip)
  - extension & abduction from flexed hip
NS - N to Obturator Internus (L5-S2)
BS - superior gluteal
T - test movements of the flexed hip to R

Occipitalis see Epicranius
Omohyoid see Thyro / Hyoid muscles

Opponens Digiti Minimi

Hypothenar eminence

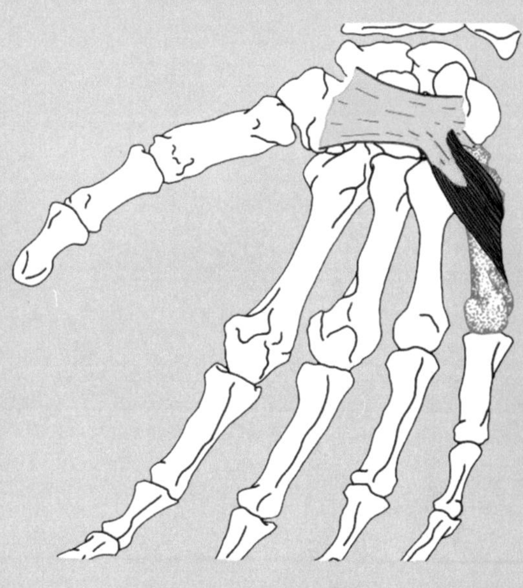

O - flexor retinaculum
  - Hamulus, Hamate
I - ulnar side of MC 5
A - flexion and apposition to thumb of little finger
NS - ulnar N deep branch (C8-T!)
BS - ulnar
T - oppose thumb and little finger with R to little finger

Opponens Pollicis
Thenar eminence

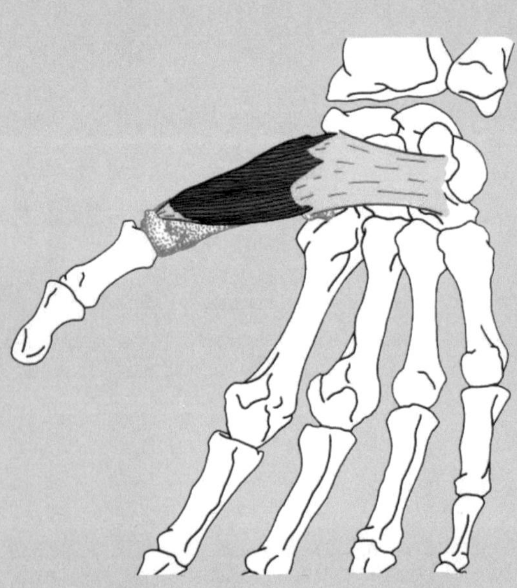

O - Trapezium (ridge)
  - flexor retinaculum
I - along the side of MC 1
A - flexion and apposition of thumb
  - adduction and medial rotation (thumb)
NS - median (C7-8)
BS - radial
T - oppose thumb and little finger with R to thumb

Orbicularis Oculi
part of the muscles of facial expression

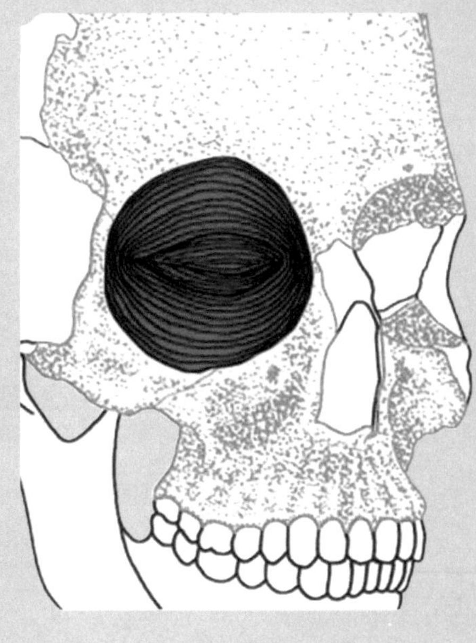

O - Frontalis, medial margin of Maxilla, Lacrimal bone
I - inserts into deep fascia of the orbit on all sides
A - closure of eyelids tightly and as in normal blinking
drainage of tear ducts
NS - facial N (CNVII)
BS - facial
T - ability to tightly close eyes

Orbicularis Oris
part of the muscles of facial expression

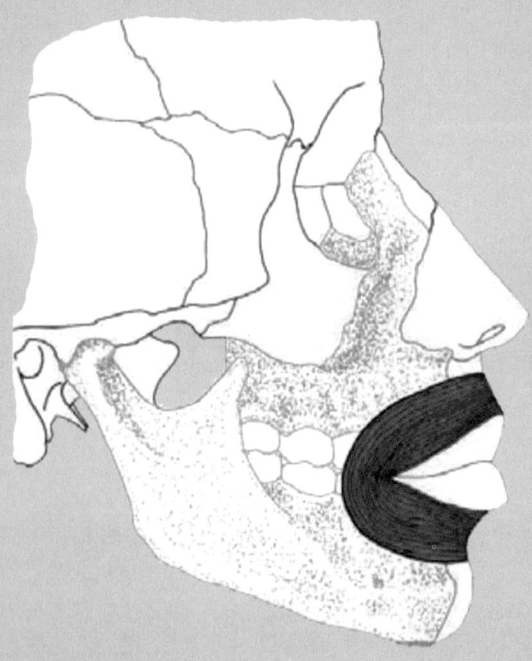

O - Maxilla,
I - deep fascia of skin and muscles around the mouth decussates extensively with the other muscles in this region
A - closure, pursing and protrusion of lips
- assists in the actions of other muscles here
NS - facial N (CN VII)
BS - facial
T - test movements of the mouth note other muscles act in synergy

Palmar Interossei

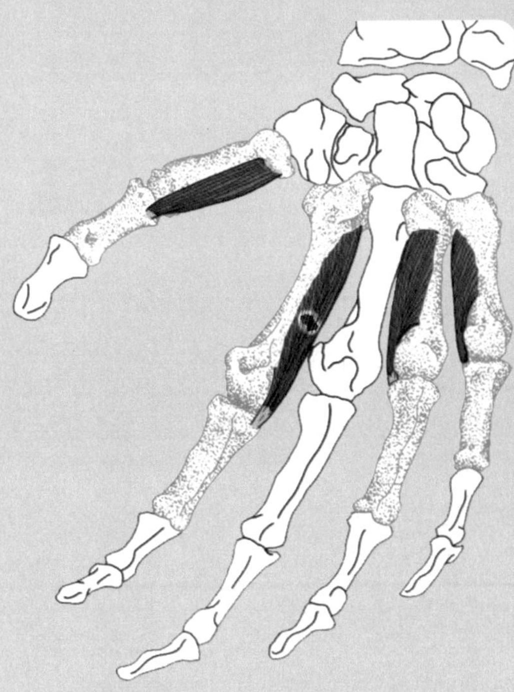

O - MCs 1-5
I - medial side of the base of the proximal Phalanges 1-2
- lateral side of the base of the proximal Phalanges 3-5
A - adduction to the middle finger
NS - ulnar N (C8-T1)
BS - deep palmer arch
T - close open fingers against R

A
B
C
D
E
F
G
H
I
J
K
L
M
N
O
P
Q
R
S
T
U
V
W
X
Y
Z

Palmaris Brevis (hand)

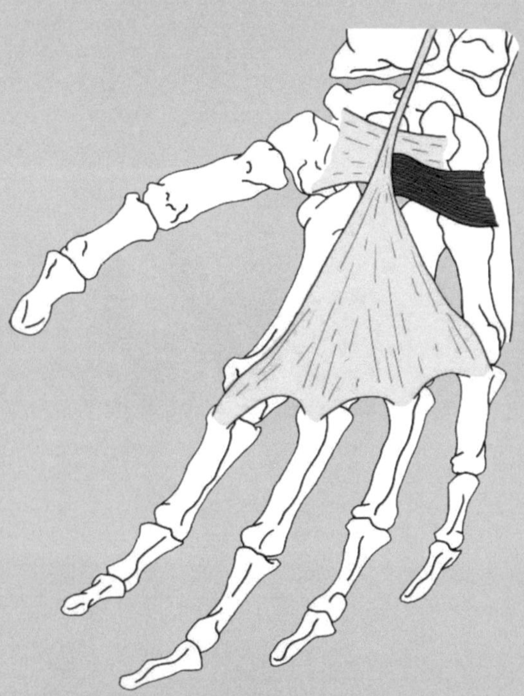

O - flexor retinaculum
- palmar aponeurosis
I - superficial fascia
A - closure of hand
NS - ulnar N (C8)
BS - superficial palmar arch
T - close open hand against R

Palmaris Longus (arm)

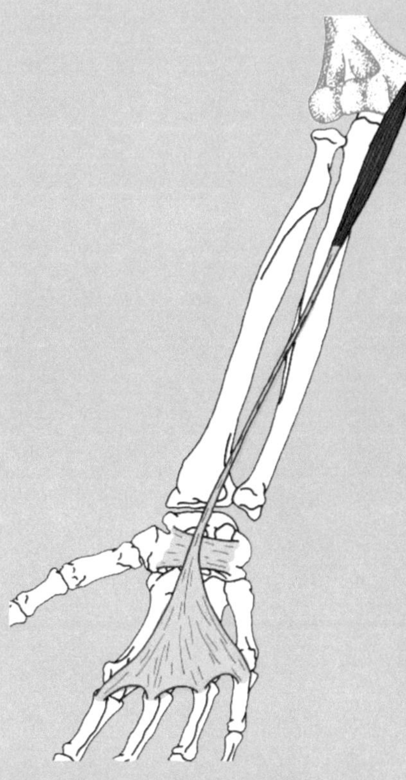

O - medial epicondyle (Humerus)
I - flexor retinaculum
- palmar aponeurosis
A - flexion of hand
NS - median N (C6-8)
BS - posterior ulnar recurrent
- superficial palmar arch
T - flex hand against R

Pectineus

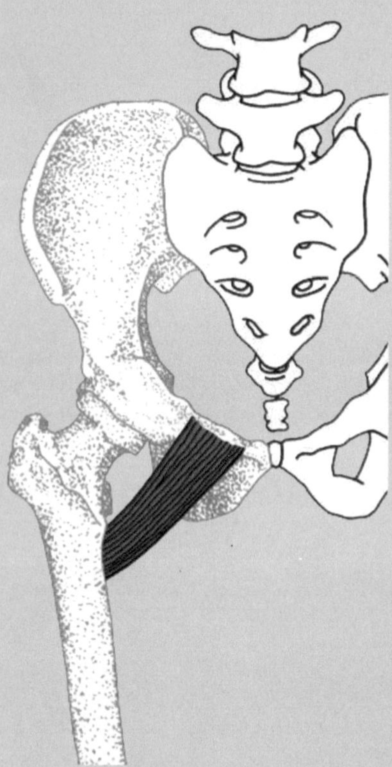

O - pubic crest & tubercle (hip)
I - upper ½ linea aspera (Femur)
A - adduction, flexion, lateral rotation (hip)
NS - femoral N (L2-4), obturator and accessory obturator Ns (L3-4)
BS - media femoral circumflex, obturator

Pectoralis Major

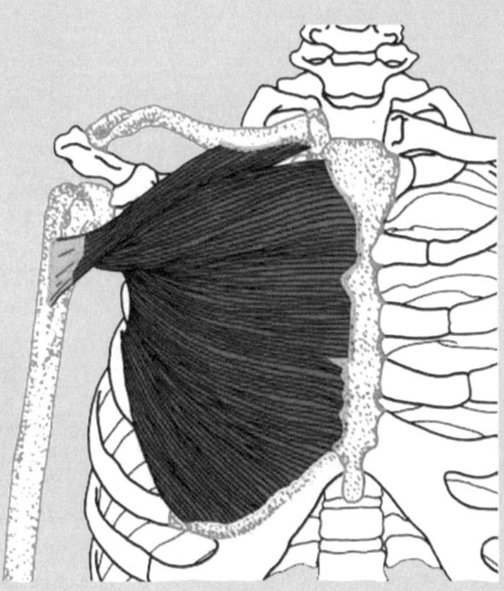

base of the breast tissue main muscle of the chest

O - medial 2/3 of the anterior clavicle
- ½ width of the anterior surface of the Sternum
- anterior surface of the cartilages of ribs 1- 6
- tendon twists over - so the clavicular fibres insert below the sternal & costal fibres

I - lateral lip of bicipital groove (Humerus)

A - fixed Sternum/chest
- adduction, horizontal adduction, medial rotation (Humerus)
- abduction > 90°
- fixed Humerus/arm (as in holding onto a fixed structure)
- accessory muscle of respiration - inspiration (eg in asthma)

NS - medial & lateral pectoral N (C5-8)

BS - thoracoacromial

T - horizontal adduction and adduction against R
- arm placed on a table moved over the surface 180° across the table to eliminate gravity

This muscle may be removed in a mastectomy if there is invasion to the deep fascia

A B C D E F G H I J K L M N O **P** Q R S T U V W X Y Z

Pectoralis Minor

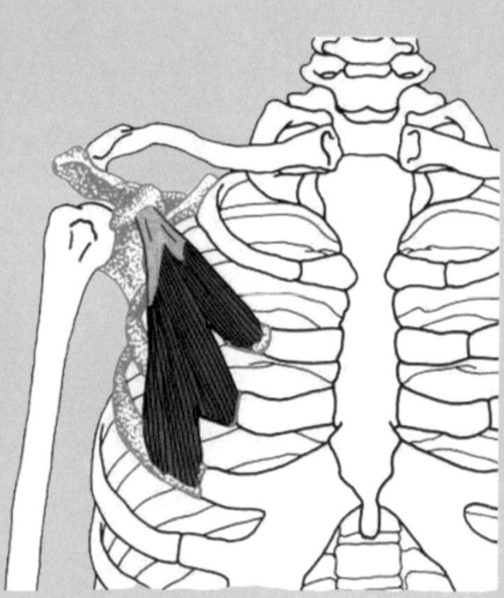

deep to Major

O - anterior surface of ribs 3-5
I - coracoid process (Scapula)
A - depression, flexion, medial rotation (shoulder)
- abduction > 90º (Humerus)
- fixed Humerus/arm (as in holding onto a fixed structure)
- accessory muscle of respiration - inspiration (eg in asthma)

NS - medial & lateral pectoral N (C5-T1)
BS - thoracoacromial
T - ability to pull their shoulders down

Peroneus Brevis
b/n Longus and Tertius

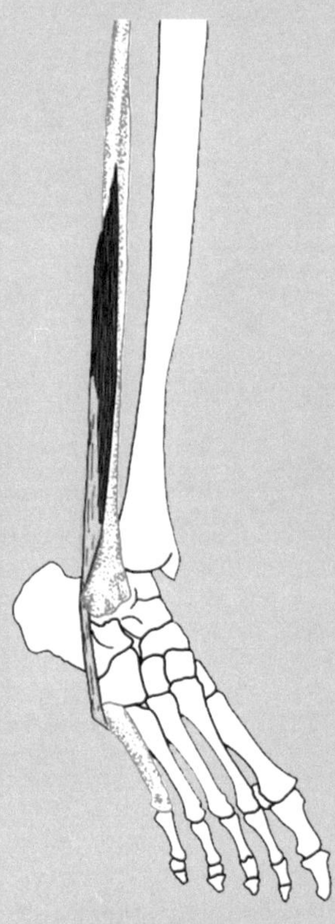

O - lower lateral surface of Fibula
I - moves beneath the foot to the base of MT1 & Cuniform1 (big toe)
A - plantar flexion (ankle)
- eversion (foot)
NS - superficial peroneal N (L5-S2)
BS - peroneal
T - plantar flex and evert against R

A
B
C
D
E
F
G
H
I
J
K
L
M
N
O
P
Q
R
S
T
U
V
W
X
Y
Z

Peroneus Longus
most superficial

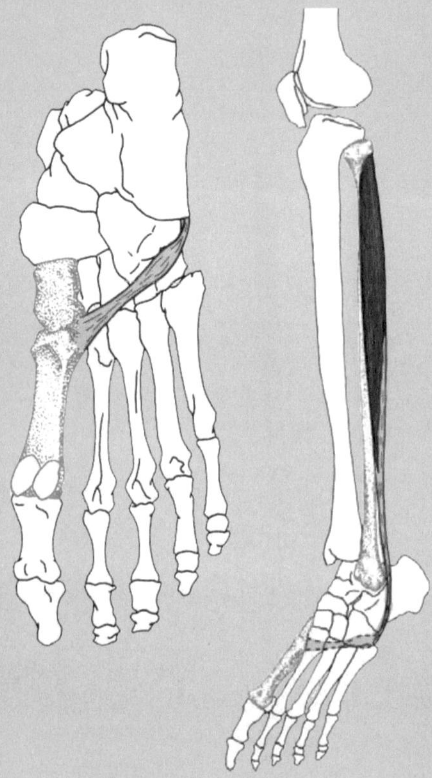

O - head, lateral surface of the Fibula
I - base of MT 5
A - plantar flexion (ankle)
- eversion (foot)
NS - superficial peroneal N (L5-S1)
BS - peroneal
T - plantar flex and evert against R

Peroneus Tertius
deepest

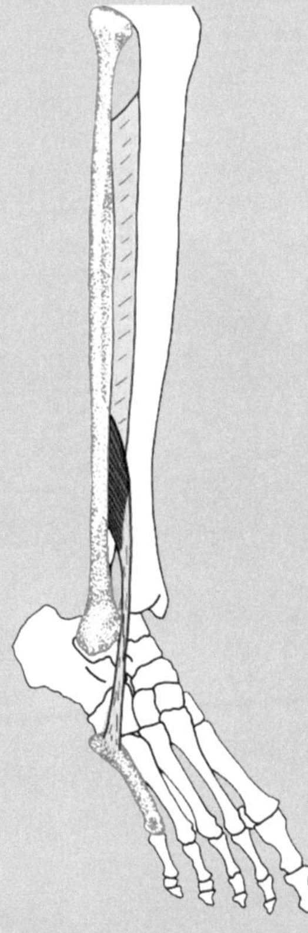

O - lower anterior of the Fibula
I - base of MT 5
A - dorsi flexion (ankle)
- eversion (foot)
NS - anterior tibial, deep peroneal N (L5-S1)
BS - anterior tibial
T - plantar flex and evert against R

A
B
C
D
E
F
G
H
I
J
K
L
M
N
O
P
Q
R
S
T
U
V
W
X
Y
Z

Piriformis

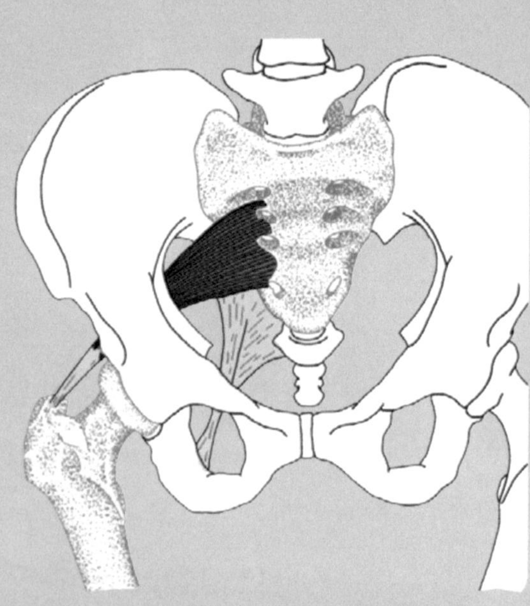

O - anterior surface of Sacrum
- sacrotuberous ligament - through the greater sciatic notch

I - superior medial surface of greater trochanter

A - lateral rotation, abduction extension (hip)

NS - inferior gluteal N (L5-S2)
- N to Piriformis from SP (S1-2)

BS - superior & inferior gluteal, internal pudendal

Important landmark for the emergence of the Sciatic N

Plantar Interossei

fourth and deepest layer of the soul

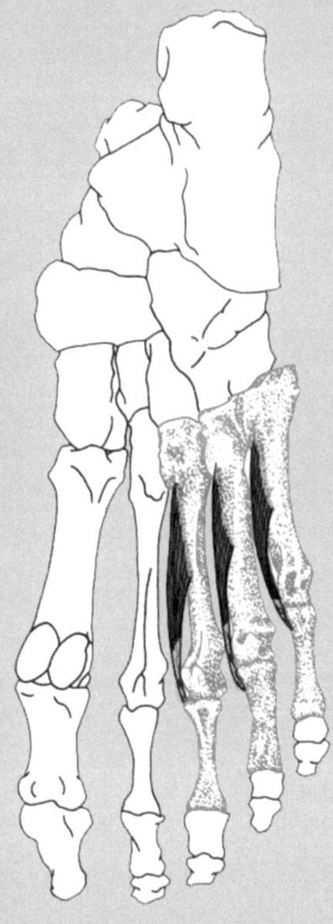

O - medial surface of MTs 3-5
I - medial surface of base Phalanx 1 Digits 3-5
A - adduction
NS - lateral plantar (superficial peroneal) N (S2-3)
BS - lateral plantar

Plantaris

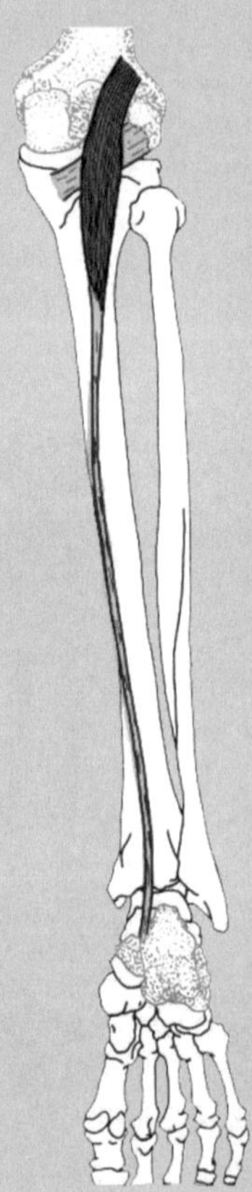

O - posterior surface of lateral condyle (Femur)
I - Calcaneal tuberosity via Achilles' tendon
A - flexion (knee)
  - dorsiflexion (ankle)
NS - medial popliteal/tibial N (L4-S1)
BS - popliteal
T - dorsiflex ankle against R

Platysma
part of the muscles of facial expression

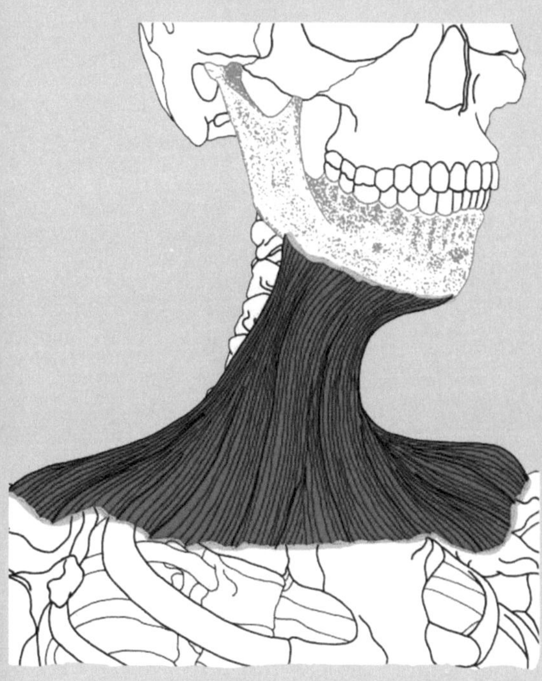

O - superficial fascia of the upper chest
I - superficial fascia of the chin and jaw up to the lower lips
A - moves the skin from lower jaw to chest
NS - facial N cervical branch (CN VII)
BS - facial, inferior alveolar, laryngeal
T - ability to tighten neck and jaw

Popliteus

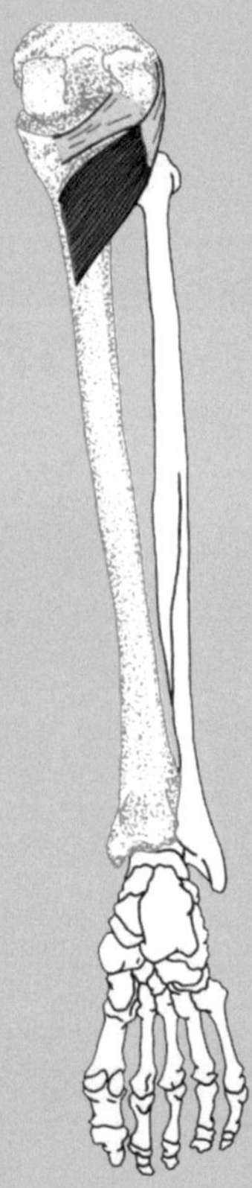

O - lateral epicondyle (Femur)
I - proximal posterior surface of Tibia
A - flexion (knee)
- medial rotation of the flexed knee
NS - medial popliteal/tibial N (L4-S1)
BS - popliteal
T - with flexed knee rotate inwards against R

Procerus - *see the summary of the muscles of the Face*

Pronator Quadratus

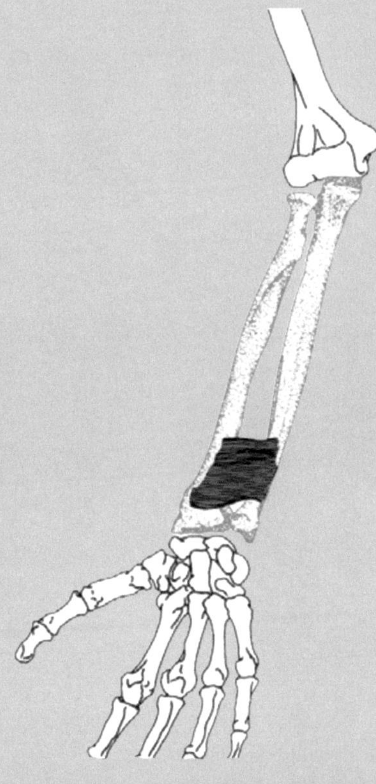

O - anterior surface of the distal ¼ of the Ulna
I - anterior surface of the distal ¼ of the Radius
A - pronation
NS - median N anterior interosseus branch (C8-T1)
BS - ulnar
T - lay arm on bench pronate against R

A B C D E F G H I J K L M N O **P** Q R S T U V W X Y Z

Pronator Teres

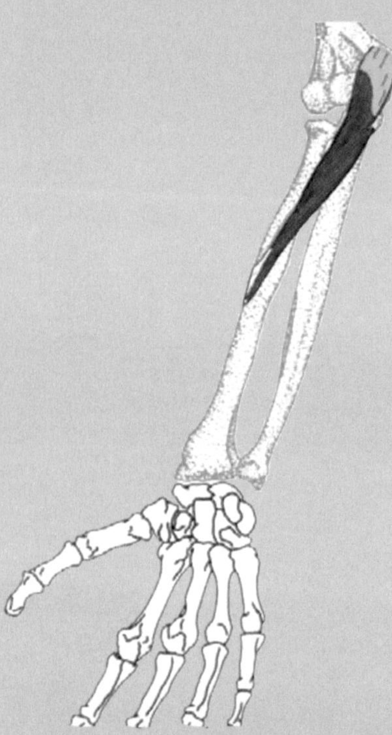

O - medial epicondyle (Humerus)
 - supracondylar ridge (Humerus)
 - coronoid process (Ulna)
I - lateral surface (Radius)
A - pronation, flexion (forearm)
NS - median N anterior interosseus branch (C6-7)
BS - anterior ulnar recurrent
T - lay extended arm on bench pronate and flex against R

Psoas

Iliopsoas = Iliacus + Psoas Major

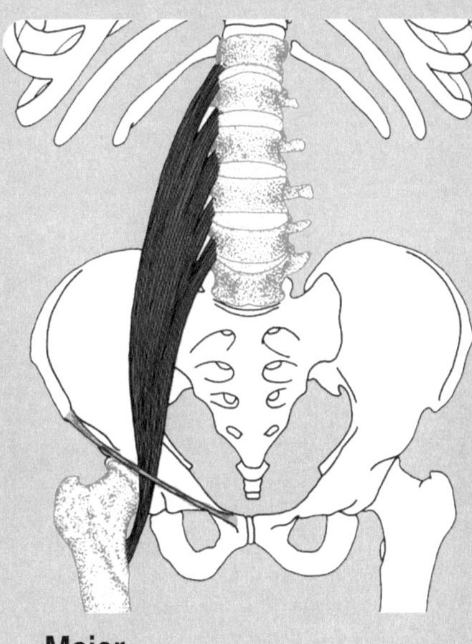

Major

completely overlays Minor and merges with Iliacus

O - bodies and TP of T12, L1-5
I - lesser trochanter (Femur)
A - flexion of hip and lower back
NS - femoral N and LP (L1-3)
BS - iliolimbar
T - ability to raise straight legs (R=gravity)

Minor

absent in 30% of patients

O - bodies and TP of L2-5
I - lesser trochanter (Femur)
A - flexion of hip and lower back
NS - femoral N and LP (L1-3)
BS - iliolimbar
T - ability to straight legs (R=gravity)

Pterygoid

part of the muscles of mastication

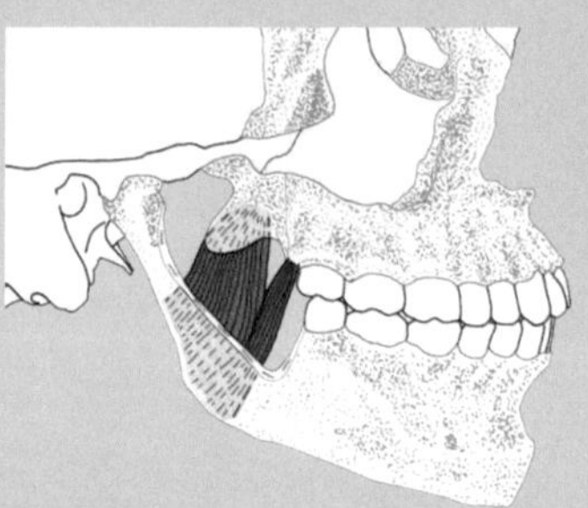

Lateral

O - superior, inferior heads, greater wing and lateral surface of the lateral pterygoid plate of Sphenoid
I - temporomandibular joint
A - opens jaw / Mandible
- moves Mandible from side to side
NS - trigeminal N (CN V)
BS - maxillary branches
T - open jaw against R

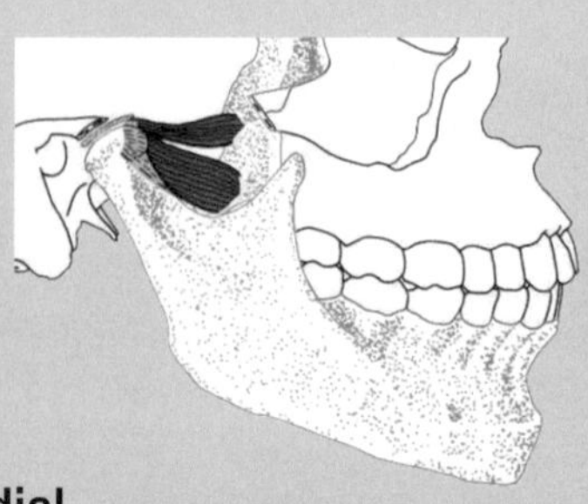

Medial

O - lateral plate of Sphenoid - lateral pterygoid plate
- Palatine bones, Maxilla
I - Mandible
A - closes jaw / Mandible
- moves Mandible back and clenches teeth
NS - trigeminal N (CN V)
BS - maxillary and its branches
T - ability to clench teeth and pull jaw back

Pyramidalis

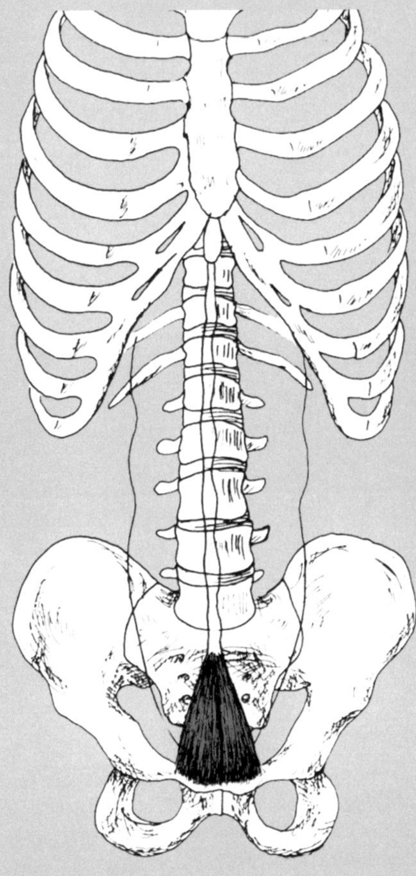

O - anterior surface of Pubic Symphysis and Pubis (pelvic ring)
I - linea alba (part of the deep fascia of the abdomen) ½ way to the umbilicus
A - compresses abdomen, supports contents
- assists in defeacation, and forced expiration
NS - subcostal N (T12)
BS - ilioinguinal, iliohypogastric
T - tighten abdomen and observe lower muscles

Quadratus Femoris

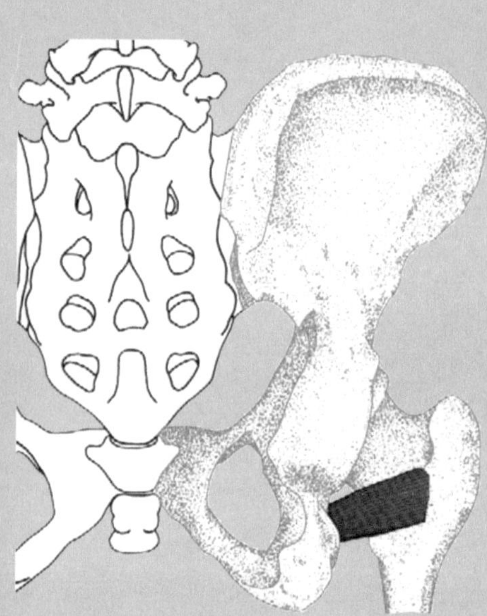

O - ischeal tubersoity (hip)
I - quadrate tubercle on intertrochanteric crest (Femur)
A - lateral rotation (Femur)
NS - N to Quadratus Femoris from SP (L4-S1)
BS - medial femoral circumflex
T - sitting on the floor legs flexed & abducted rotate legs outwards

Quadratus Lumborum

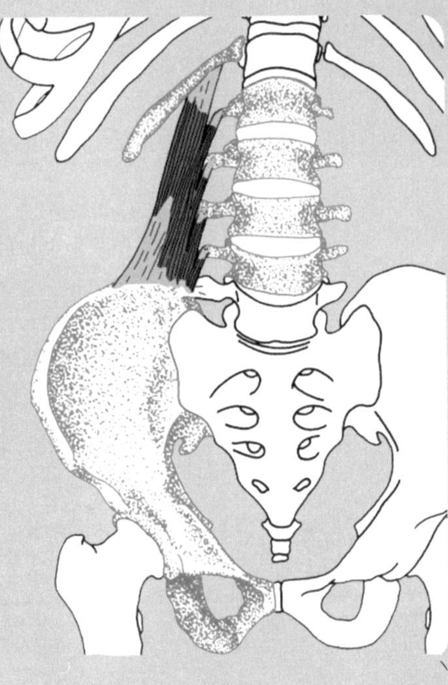

O - posterior crest of Ileum (hip)
I - rib 12, TP of L1-5
A - bilateral = lumbar extension (lower back)
- unilateral = lateral flexion (lower back)
- augments action of Diaphragm,
- supports lower back
- supports abdominal & pelvic contents (core muscle)
NS - subcostal N, LP (T12-L3)
BS - lumbar vessels
T - erect standing patient bends to the side
- hyperextension of lower back - care needed with some patients

Quadratus Plantae

2nd layer soul of the foot

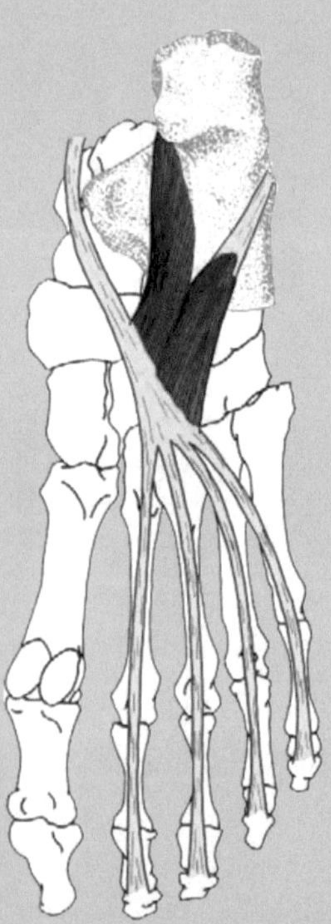

O - 2 heads medial, lateral
- medial medial inferior surface of Calcaneus
- lateral lateral surface Calcaneus, long plantar ligament

I - tendon of Flexor Digitorum Longus

A - plantar flexion

NS - lateral plantar N (L4-S2)

BS - lateral plantar

T - foot, plantar flexion against R
- observation of arch and changes with flexion

Rectus Abdominis

Segmental muscles 4-5 divisions - often asymmetric

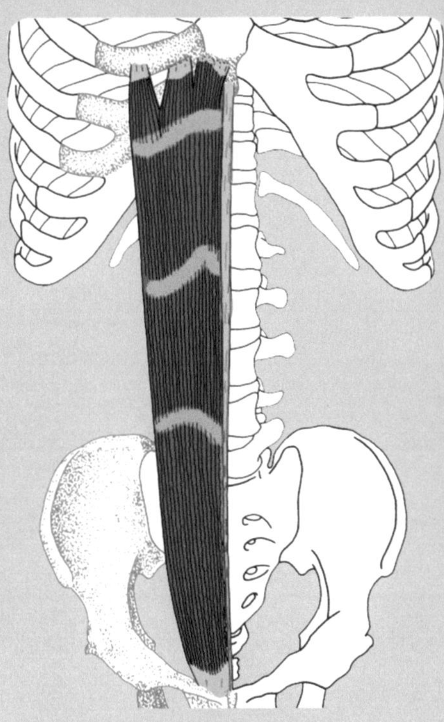

O - anterior surface of Pubic Symphysis and crest of Pubis (hips pelvic ring)

I - xiphoid process (Sternum)
 - costal cartilages ribs 5-7

A - bilateral - lateral flexion and flexion of trunk/abdomen, supports contents
 - assists in defeacation
 - unilateral - rotation of abdomen

NS - subcostal N (T12), lower intercostal Ns (T5-12)

BS - inferior epigastric, lower intercostals

T - tense and bend abdomen - sit ups

Rectus Capitis

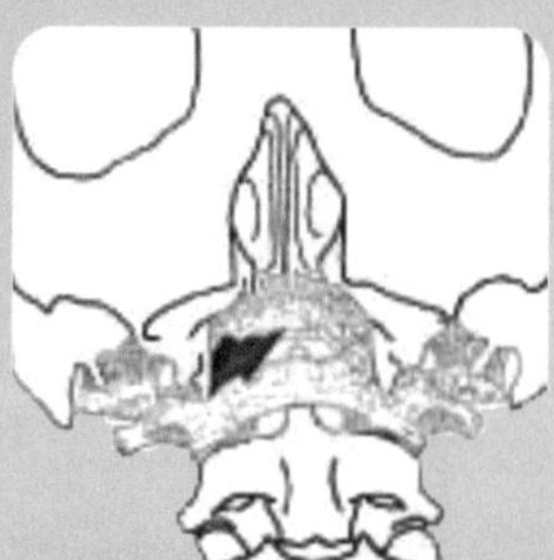

Anterior

O - TP of Atlas (C1)
I - Occiput - inferior surface of basilar part
A - flexion (head)
NS - N to Rectus Capitus part of CP (C2-3), suboccipital N (C1)
BS - vertebral
T - flex head against R

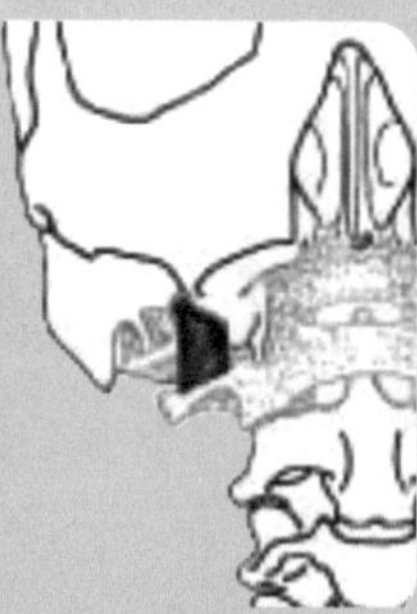

Lateralis

O - TP of Atlas (C1)
I - Occiput - jugular process
A - lateral flexion (head) unilateral action
NS - N to Rectus Lateralis (C1-3) part of CP
BS - vertebral
T - laterally flex head against R

Rectus Capitis

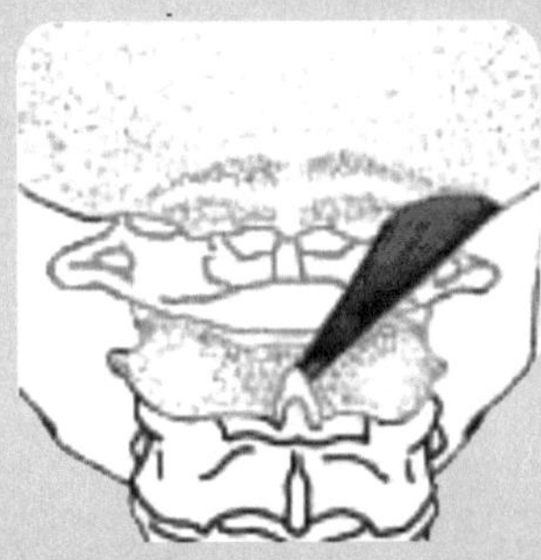

Posterior - Major

O - SP of Axis (C2)
I - Occiput - lateral ½ of inferior nuchal line
A - bilateral extension (head)
- unilateral ipsi-rotation - (to the same side)
NS - suboccipital N (C1)
BS - vertebral, occipital
T - extend head against R

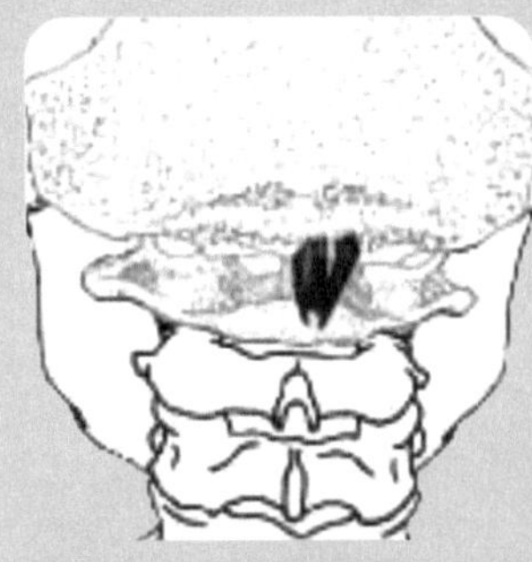

Posterior - Minor

O - posterior arch of Atlas (C1)
I - Occiput - medial ½ of the inferior nuchal line
A - extension (head)
NS - suboccipital N (C1)
BS - vertebral, occipital
T - extend head against R

Rectus Femoris

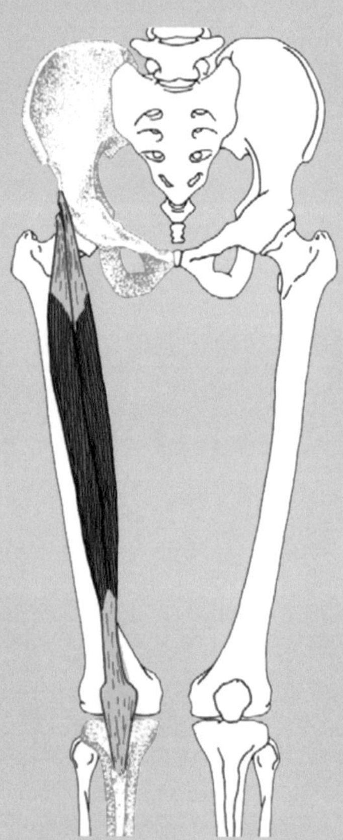

O - ASIS (hip)
I - quadratus tendon through to tibial tuberosity
A - flexion (hip) - stabilizes the hip
  - extension (knee)
NS - femoral N (L2-4)
BS - lateral femoral circumflex
T - sitting patient extend knee against R

Rhomboideus Major (Major Rhomboid)

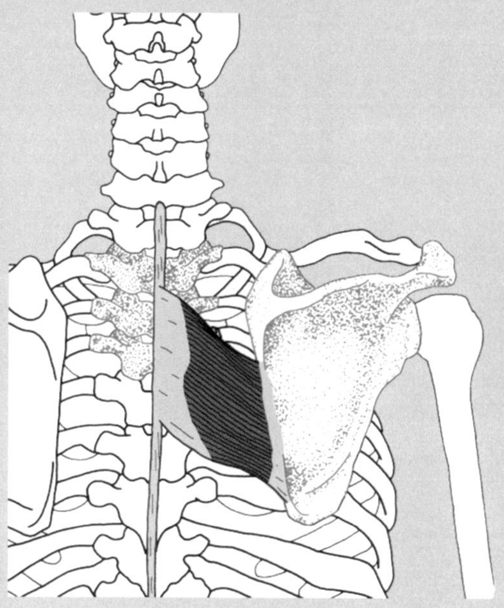

O - SP of C7-T5
I - inferior angle of medial border and spine of Scapula
A - elevation, medial rotation (shoulders/shoulder blade)
- adduction (arm via shoulder blade)
NS - dorsal scapular N (C4-5)
BS - transverse cervical

Rhomboideus Minor

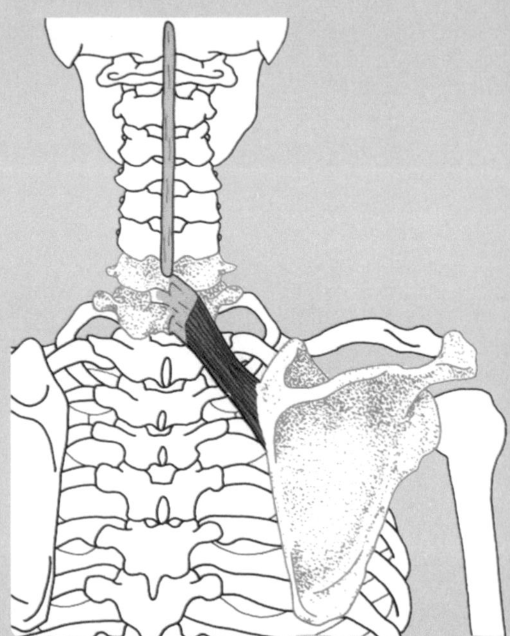

O - SP of C7-T1
I - inferior angle of medial border and spine of Scapula
A - elevation, medial rotation (shoulders/shoulder blade)
- adduction (arm via shoulder blade)
NS - dorsal scapular N (C4)
BS - transverse cervical

Risorius

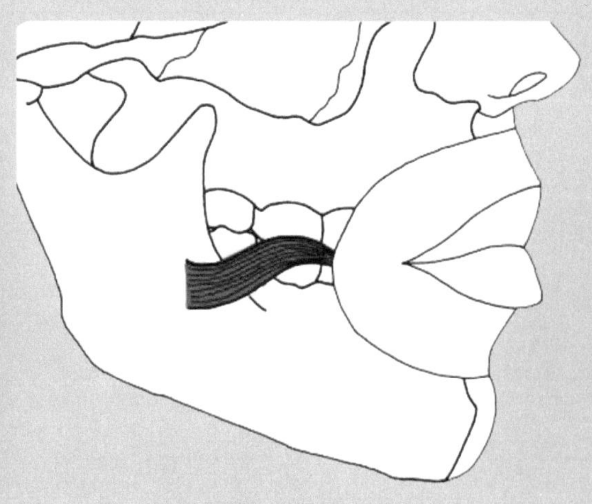

O - deep fascia of the face superficial to Masseter
I - skin at the angle of the mouth
A - grinning (variable)
NS - facial N (CN VII)
BS - facial - transverse branch
T - ability to smile "wryly"

A B C D E F G H I J K L M N O P Q **R** S T U V W X Y Z

Rotatores

part of the deepest layer of muscles of the Spine - VC series of small muscles extending from Atlas to Sacrum Longus completely overlays Brevis

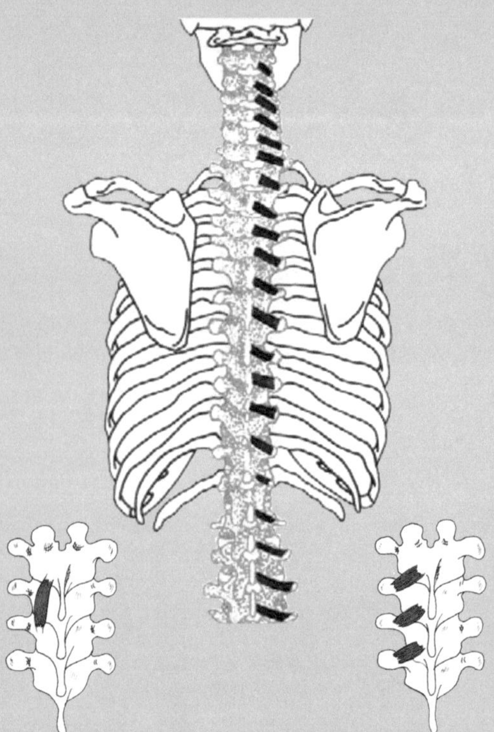

O&I - Longus - SP to lamina of the VB 2 above
- Brevis - SP to lamina of the VB 1 above

A - bilateral - extension of the VC
- unilateral - rotation of the VC at the level of individual VBs

NS - segmental dorsal rami of the SNs

BS - segmental dorsal branches of the local vessels eg intercostals, iliolumbar etc

Salpingopharyngeus - *see the Pharyngeal Muscles*

Sartorius

part of anterior compartment of the thigh

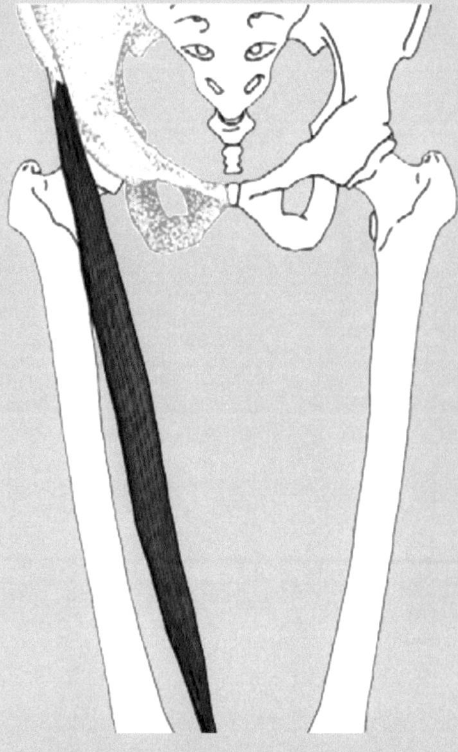

O - ASIS of hip
I - anteriomedial surface of Tibia
A - flexion (hip and knee)
- abduction & lateral rotation (hip)
NS - femoral N (L4-5)
BS - femoral
T - patient lying on the side with flexed hip and extended leg from here ability to flex knee against R (gravity eliminated)

A B C D E F G H I J K L M N O P Q R **S** T U V W X Y Z

Scalenus Anterior, Medial & Posterior

Scalene muscles

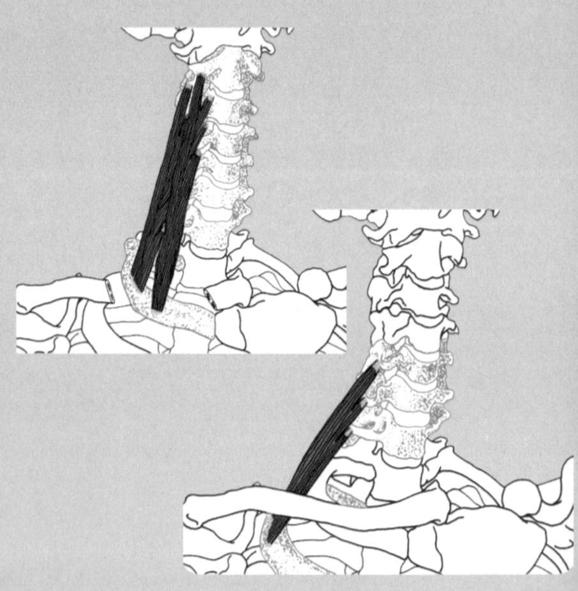

O - Anterior TP of C3-7
- Medial TP of C3-7
- Posterior TP of C5-7

I - Anterior anteromedial surface of rib 1
- Medial lateral to the anterior muscle rib 1
- Posterior rib 2 inferior to the Clavicle

A - elevation of the ribs for unilateral action ll muscles
- in forced inspiration
- bilateral - flexion (neck)
- unilateral - rotation & lateral flexion of the neck

NS - segmental - SNs anterior branches (C4-7 anterior & lateral C6-8 posterior) supraclavicular branches of the BP Ns (C4-8) N to Longus Colli and N to Scaleni muscles

BS - superficial cervical

T - flex neck against R
- laterally flex neck against R

Semimembranosus

part of Hamstrings - posterior compartment of the thigh

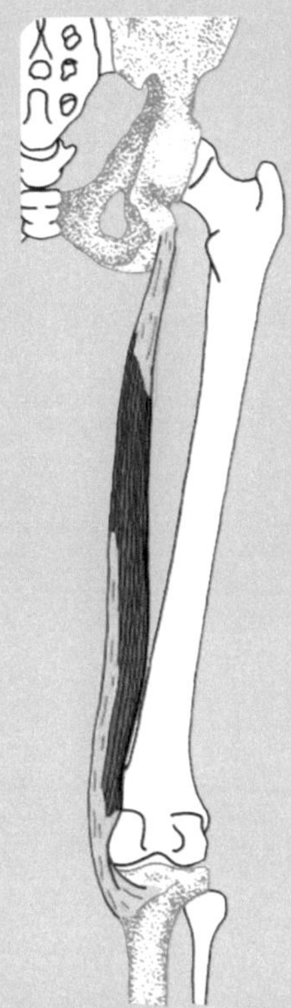

O - ischeal tuberosity (hip)
I - posterior surface of the medial condyle (Tibia)
A - extension (hip)
- flexion (knee)
- lateral rotation (flexed knee)
NS - sciatic N (L5-S2)
BS - deep femoral
T - patient lying on the side with flexed hip and extended leg ability to draw up both hip and knee against R (gravity eliminated)

Semispinalis

part of the deep muscles of the spine / neck more lateral than Spinalis

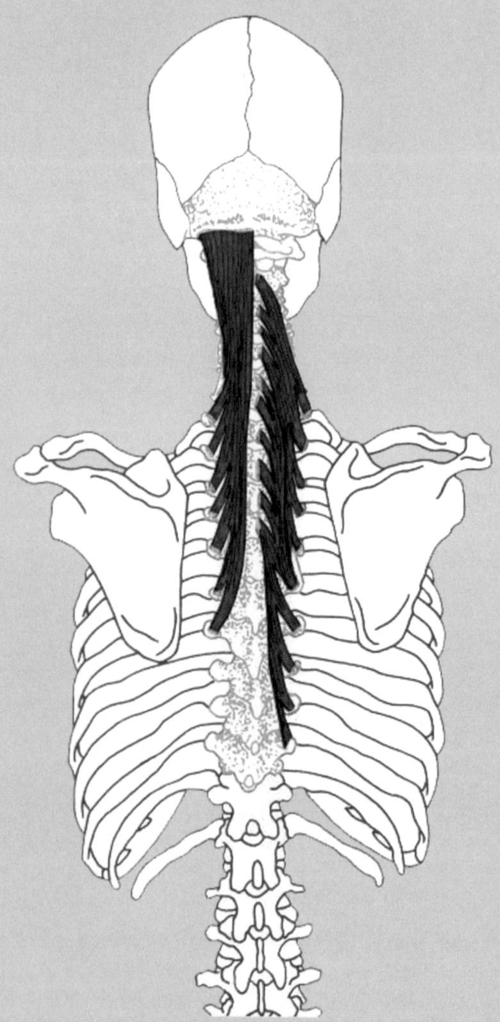

Capitis

O - TP of C4-7
I - superior & inferior nuchal lines (Occiput)
A - bilateral extension (head)
- unilateral rotation (head)
NS - suboccipital N - dorsal rami (C1)

Cervicis

O - TP of T1-6
I - SP of C1-5
A - bilateral extension (neck)
- unilateral rotation (head)
NS - dorsal rami of the segmental SNs (C2-T5)

Thoracis

O - TP of T6-10
I - SP of C6-T4
A - bilateral extension (thorax)
- unilateral rotation (thorax)
NS - dorsal branches of the segmental SNs (C5-T11)
BS - segmental branches from local BVs
T - ability to extend back in a prone position and extend and rotate neck

A B C D E F G H I J K L M N O P Q R **S** T U V W X Y Z

Semitendinosus

part of Hamstrings - posterior compartment of the thigh

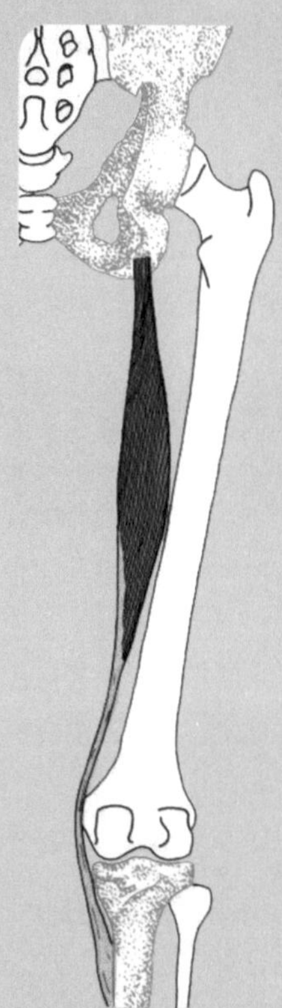

O - ischeal tuberosity (hip)
I - medial surface of the proximal shaft of the Tibia
A - flexion (knee)
 - medial rotation (flexed knee)
NS - sciatic N (L5-S2)
BS - deep femoral
T - ability of the standing patient to rotate knee inwards

Serratus Anterior

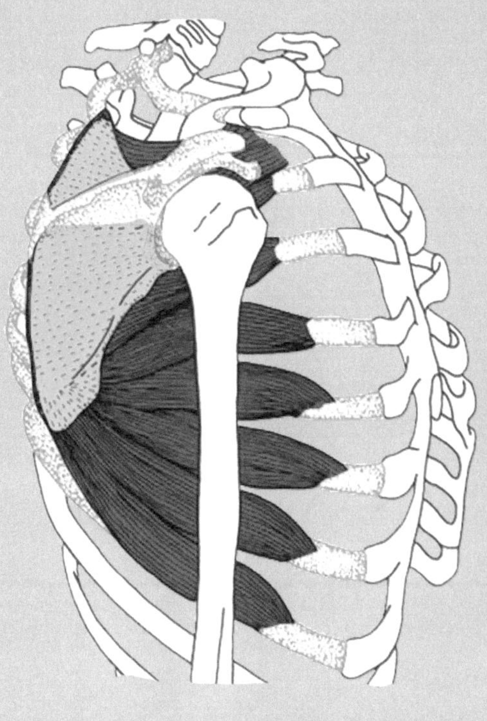

O - lateral surface of ribs 1-9
I - costal surface of the vertebral boarder of the Scapula
A - abduction (Scapula - shoulder)
- lateral rotation (shoulder - pulling shoulders back
- fixed upper limb accessory breathing muscle - inspiration
- protraction (drawing shoulders down)
NS - long thoracic (C5-7)
BS - lateral thoracic
T - ability to pull down shoulders and arms

Serratus Posterior

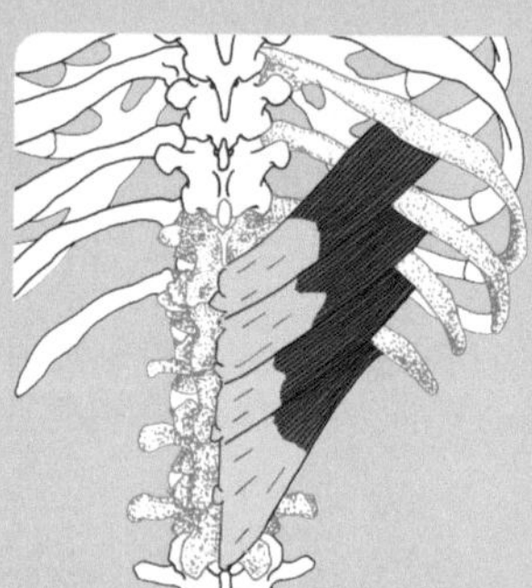

Inferior

O - SP of T11-L3
I - lateral surface of ribs 8-12
A - pulls ribs downwards (for expiration)
NS - lower intercostal Ns, subcostal N (T7-12)
BS - intercostals, iliohypogastric
T - forced expiration w/o assistance from accessory muscles observe lower rib movement

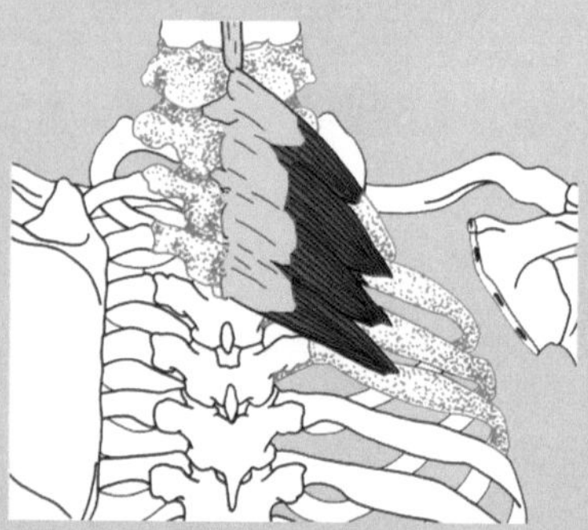

Superior

O - ligamentum nuchae
- SP of C1-T3
I - lateral surface to angle of ribs 2-5
A - pulls ribs upwards (for inspiration)
NS - upper intercostal Ns (T1-4)
BS - intercostal BVs
T - observation of the upper ribs in inspiration

Soleus

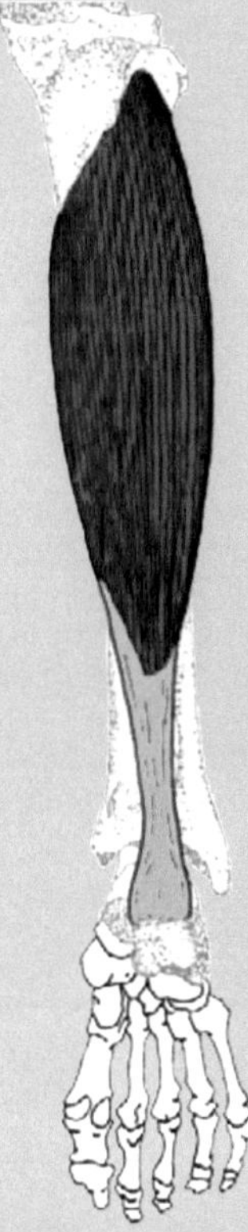

O - upper shaft, posterior surface (Tibia & Fibula)
I - Achille's tendon to tuberosity of Calcaneus
A - plantar flexion (foot)
NS - medial popliteal, tibial N (S1-2)
BS - posterior tibial
- peroneal
- popliteal
T - ability of the standing patient to go on their toes

Sphincter Ani - External Anal Sphincter

sphincter hence circular muscle inserting all around natural position - constricted rather than relaxed

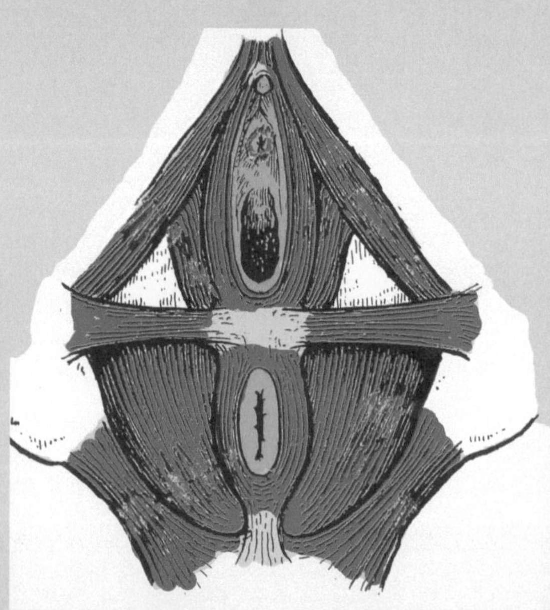

O - submuscosa of the rectum extending to deep fascia of the skin
I - peroneal body
  - fibres of Levator Ani
A - relaxation causes release of rectal contents
NS - inferior rectal Ns from SP (S2-4)
   - pudendal N (S2-4)
BS - inferior rectal vessels
   - haemorrhoidal vessels
T - faecal continence

Sphincter Urethrae - Urethral Sphincter

sphincter hence circular muscle inserting all around
natural position - constricted rather than relaxed

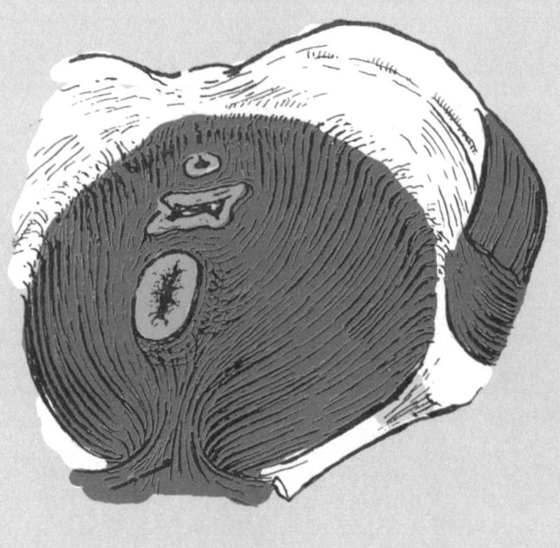

O - submuscosa of the urethra
I - peroneal diaphragm
- in females - anterior wall of the vagina
A - relaxation causes release of bladder contents
NS - pudendal N (S2-4)
BS - inferior vaginal vessels
- branches from internal iliacs
- pudendal vessels
T - urinary continence

Spinalis

part of ES

more medial than and superficial to Semispinalis

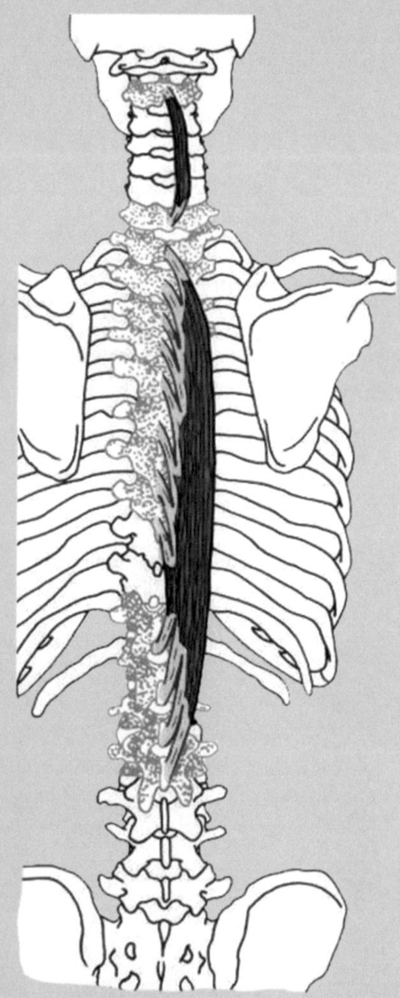

Capitus

O - TP of C4-7
I - superior nuchal lines (Occiput)
A - bilateral extension (head and upper VC)
- unilateral rotation (head and neck)
NS - dorsal branches of SN - dorsal rami (C1-8)

Cervicis

O - ligamentum nuchae
- SP of C7
I - SP of C1
A - bilateral extension (upper VC)
- unilateral stabilization (neck)
NS - dorsal rami of the segmental SNs (C2-8)

Spinalis Thoracis

O - TP of T11-L2
I - SP of T1-8
A - bilateral extension (thorax)
- unilateral stabilization of thorax
NS - dorsal branches of the segmental SNs (T9-L2)
BS - segmental branches from local BVs

T - ability to extend back in a prone position and extend neck

Splenius
superficial to Spinalis

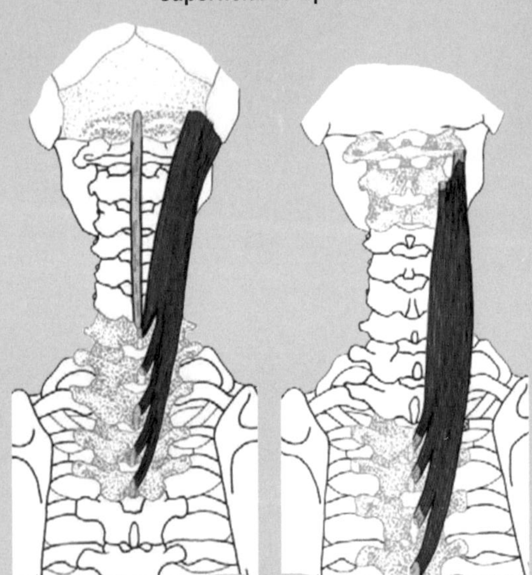

Capitus
O - TP of T1-3
I - superior nuchal lines (Occiput)
- lateral mastoid process (Temporal bone)
A - bilateral hyperextension, extension (head and neck)
- stabilization (head)
- unilateral rotation (head and neck)
NS - dorsal branches of SN - dorsal rami (C1-2)
- suboccipital N, greater occipital N (C1-2)

Cervicis
O - ligamentum nuchae and TP of C1-3
I - SP and interspinous ligaments of T1-4
A - bilateral extension, hyperextension (neck and upper VC)
- unilateral stabilization (neck)
NS - dorsal rami of the segmental SNs (C3-8)
BS - branches of the internal carotids
T - ability to hyper-extend the head and neck

Sternocleidomastoid

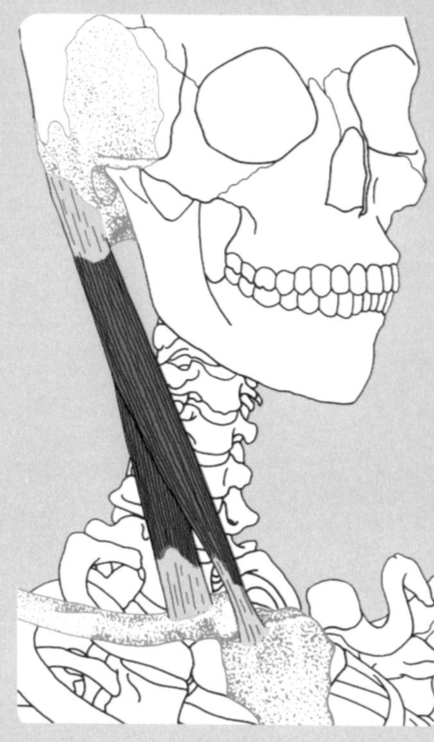

O - Manubrium (breastbone)
  - anterior surface of medial 1/3 of the Clavicle
I - mastoid process (Temporal bone)
A - bilateral flexion (head and neck)
  - unilateral rotation (head and neck)
NS - accessory N (CN XI)
  - N to Sternocleidomastoid (ventral rami of SNs C1-2)
BS - superficial cervical
T - turn head against R
  - flex head against R

Sternohyoid - *see Thyro / Hyoid Muscles*
Sternothyoid - *see Thyro / Hyoid Muscle*
Stylopharyngeus - *see Pharyngeal Muscles*

Subclavius

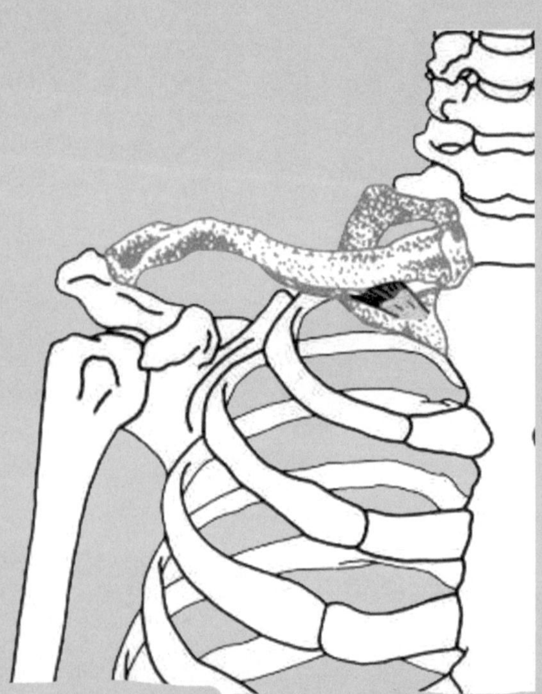

O - anterosuperior surface of rib 1
I - inferior groove on the Clavicle
A - depression of Clavicle
- stabilizer of sternoclavicular joint
NS - N to Subclavius (C5-6) from branches of BP
BS - superficial cervical
- thoracoacromial

Subcostales

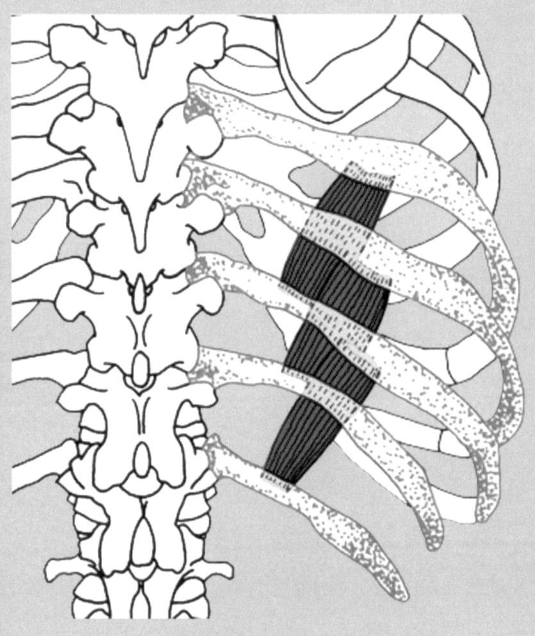

O - angle of the ribs 1-10
I - medial end of 2-3 ribs inferior - below
A - forced expiration
NS - intercostal Ns T1-12
BS - intercostal BVs
T - observe the extent of unassisted forced expiration

A B C D E F G H I J K L M N O P Q R **S** T U V W X Y Z

Subscapularis

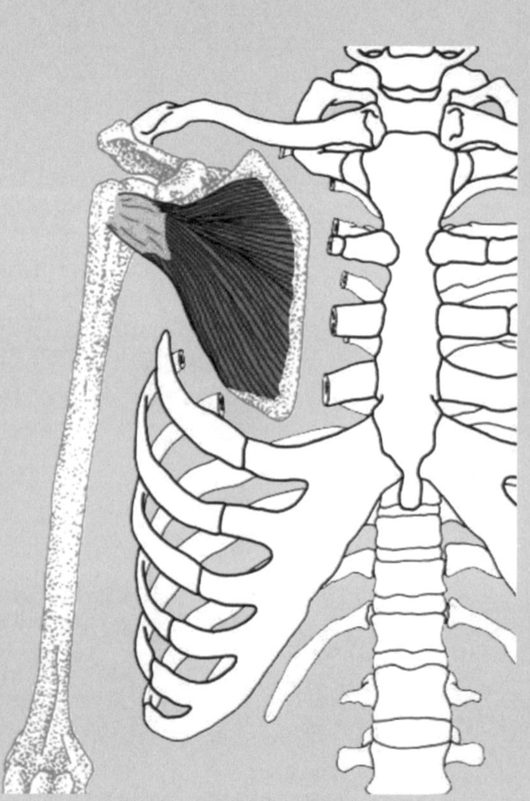

O - subscapular fossa (Scapula)
I - lesser tuberosity (Humerus)
A - medial rotation (arm)
  - adduction
NS - upper and lower subscapular Ns (C5-7)
BS - lateral thoracic
  - subscapular
T - turn arm inwards against R

Supinator

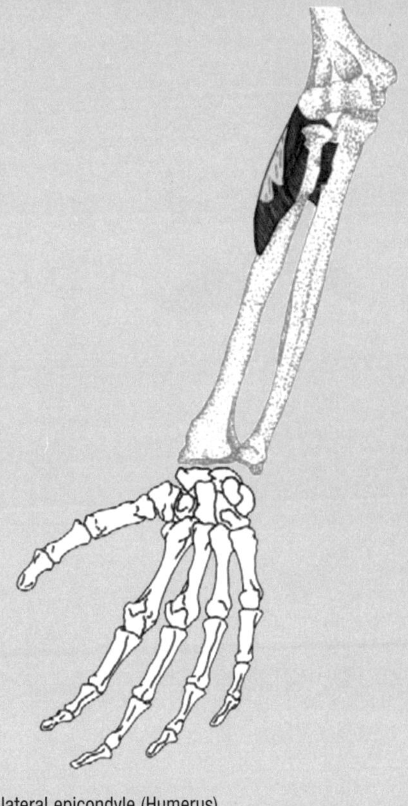

O - lateral epicondyle (Humerus)
  - collateral radial ligament
  - annular ligament
  - crest (Ulna)
I - proximal 1/3 of Radius
A - supination (forearm)
  - medial rotation (arm)
NS - radial N, deep radial & posterior interosseus branches (C5-6)
BS - radial
T - supination of forearm against R

Superior Pharyngeal Constrictor - *see Pharyngeal Constrictors*

Supraspinatus

Part of the rotator cuff muscles of the shoulder

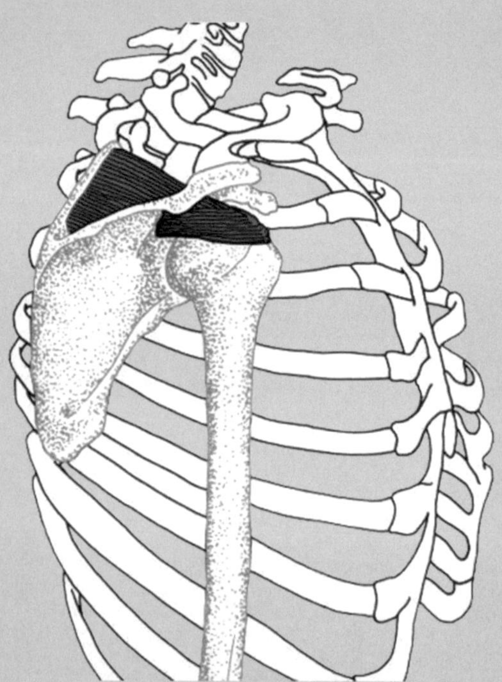

O - supraspinous fossa (Scapula)
I - greater tuberosity (Humerus)
  - shoulder joint capsule
A - draws head of Humerus up into the shoulder
  - abduction > 180º (arm)
  - stabilizer of shoulder joint
NS - suprascapular N (C4-6)
BS - suprascapular
  - axillary
T - hyperextension of arm > 180º against R

Temporalis

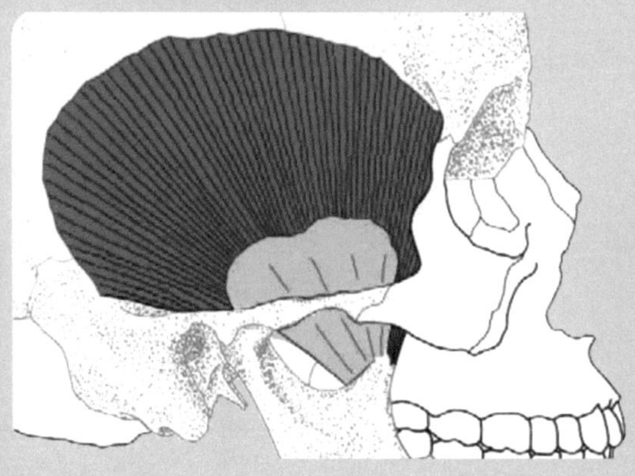

O - temporal fossa of the Frontal, Parietal and Temporal bone
I - coronoid process and ramus (Mandible)
A - closes jaw
- retracts Mandible
- clenches teeth
NS - trigeminal N (CNV)
BS - maxillary
- middle & superior temporals
T - test strength of closed jaw or close against R (with care)

Tensor Fascia Lata

part of the Iliotibial tract - lateral compartment of the thigh

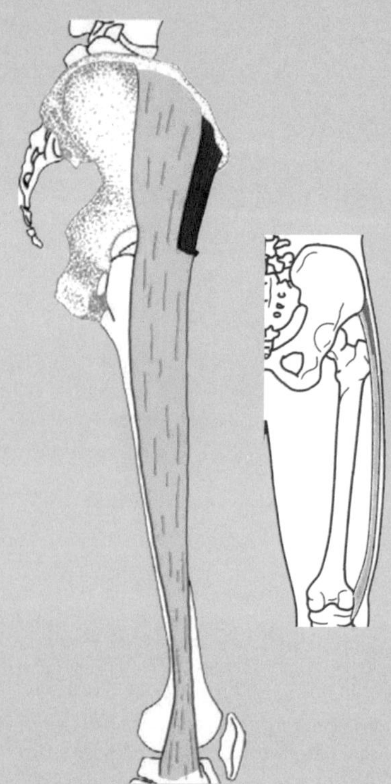

O - anterior iliac crest (Ileum –hip)
I - iliotibial tract
A - flexion, abduction & medial rotation (Femur on hip)
NS - superior gluteal (L4-S1)
BS - superior gluteal
- lateral femoral circumflex
T - patient to abduct leg when standing R = gravity
- supine patient to abduct leg against R

Tensor Veli Palatini - *see Soft Palate Muscles*

Teres Major

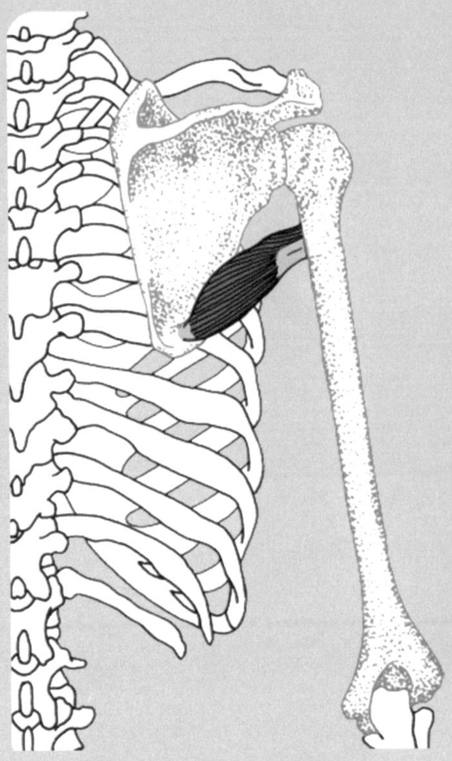

O - lower posterio-lateral border of Scapula
I - medial lip of the bicipital groove (Humerus)
A - extension, medial rotation (shoulder)
 - horizontal abduction (shoulder)
NS - lower subscapular N (C5-7)
BS - scapular circumflex

Teres Minor

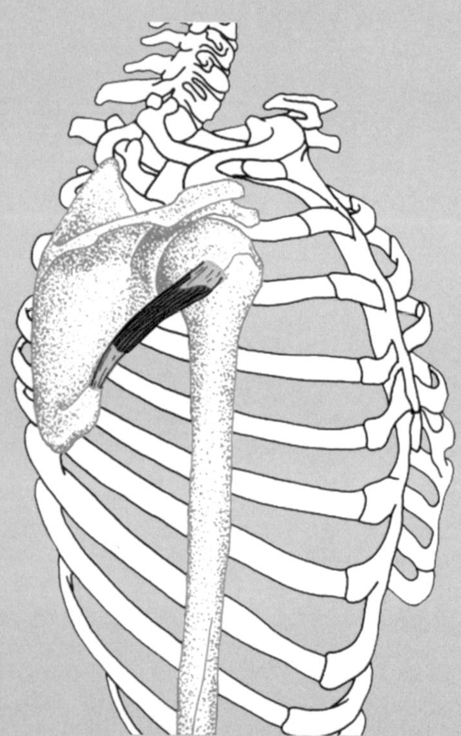

O - lower posterio-lateral border of Scapula
I - inferior surface of greater tuberosity (Humerus)
A - lateral rotation (shoulder)
  - horizontal abduction (shoulder)
NS - axillary N (C4-5)
BS - scapular circumflex
T - patient with arm resting on table move in an horizontal arc away from sagittal plane against R

Thyrohyoid - *see Thyro / Hyoid Muscles*

Tibialis Anterior

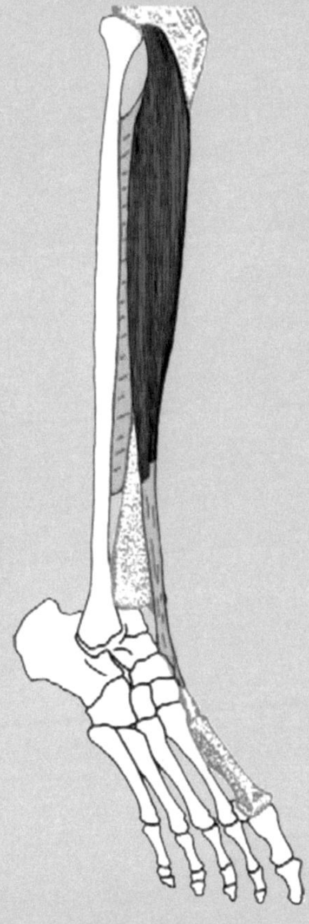

O - lateral tibial surface
I - base of MT 1
A - dorsiflexion (ankle)
  - inversion (foot)
NS - anterior tibial N, deep peroneal N (L4-S1)
BS - anterior tibial
T - invert foot against R
  - dorsiflex foot against R

Tibialis Posterior

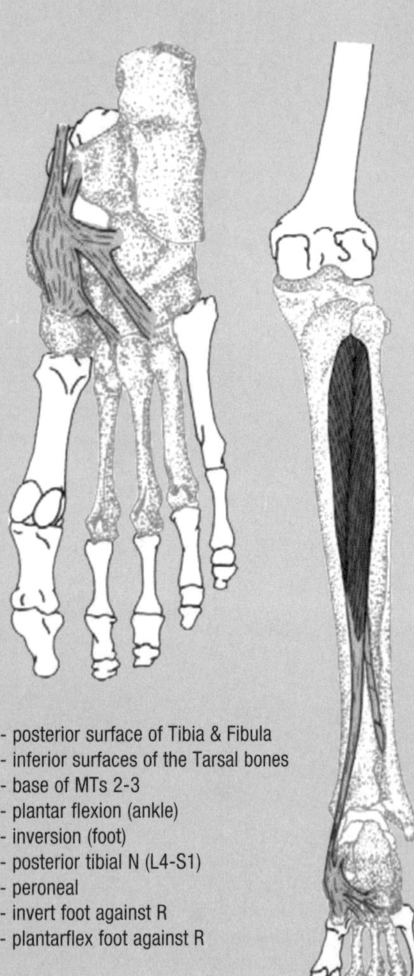

O - posterior surface of Tibia & Fibula
I - inferior surfaces of the Tarsal bones
  - base of MTs 2-3
A - plantar flexion (ankle)
  - inversion (foot)
NS - posterior tibial N (L4-S1)
BS - peroneal
T - invert foot against R
  - plantarflex foot against R

Transversus Abdominis
deepest layer of the abdominal wall

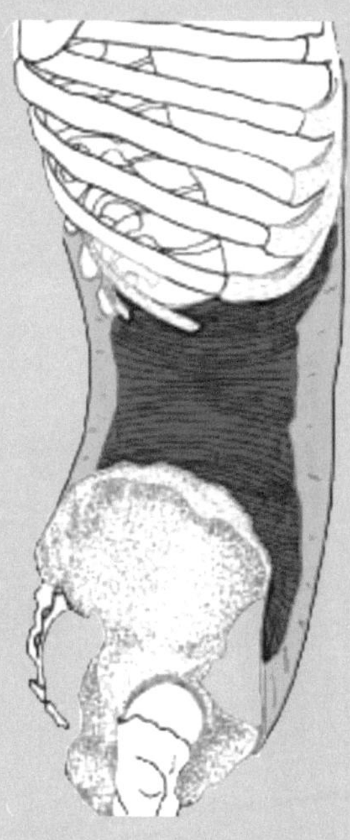

O - costal cartilages of lower ribs (7-12)
- lumbar fascia
- crest of Ileum (hip)

I - linea alba

A - compresses abdomen
- helps with defeacation
- helps with forced expiration - diaphragm
- stabilizes VC - core muscle

NS - segmental intercostal Ns (T7-12)
- iliohypogastric, ilioinguinal & subcostal Ns (T12-L1)

BS - iliolumbar
- deep iliac circumflex

T - ability to pull in the waist

Transverse Perineal - Profundus, Superficialis
- see the muscles of the Pelvis and Perineum

Trapezius upper, middle, lower

Most superficial muscle of the back

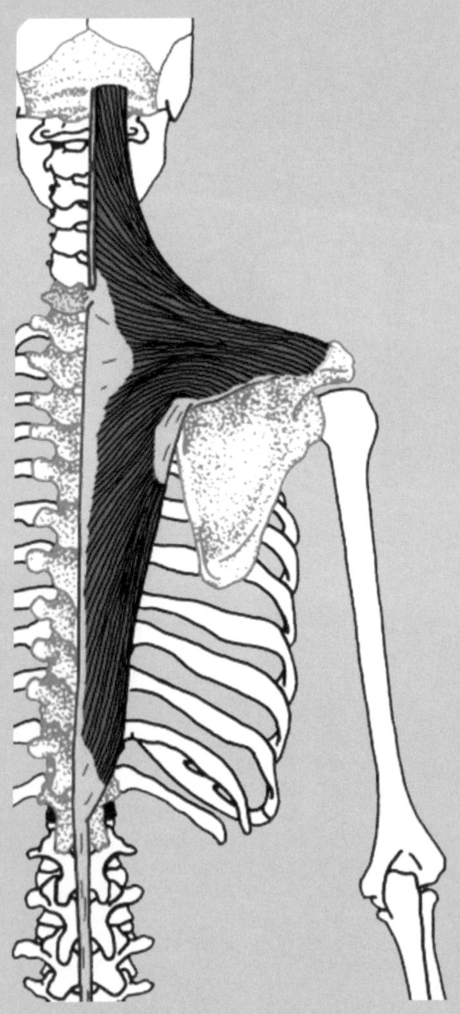

O - external occipital protuberance (skull)
- medial 1/3 superior nuchal line (Occiput)
- ligamentum nuchae
- SP of C7, T1-12 & their supra-, inter-, spinous ligaments

I - lateral 1/3 of the Clavicle
- medial border of acromion (Scapula)
- spine of Scapula

A - elevation, upward rotation - upper fibres (Scapula)
- extension, adduction - middle fibres (Scapula)
- depression, downward rotation - lower fibres (Scapula)

NS - accessory N (CN XI) - upper, middle fibres
- ventral rami of C3-4 = N to Trapezius - upper, middle fibres
- dorsal roots C1-5 - lower fibres

BS - transverse cervical
- segmental - dorsal branches of intercostals

T - elevation of shoulder blades - upper, middle fibres (against R)
- depression of shoulder blades - lower fibres

Triceps Brachii

3 headed muscle - long, lateral & medial heads

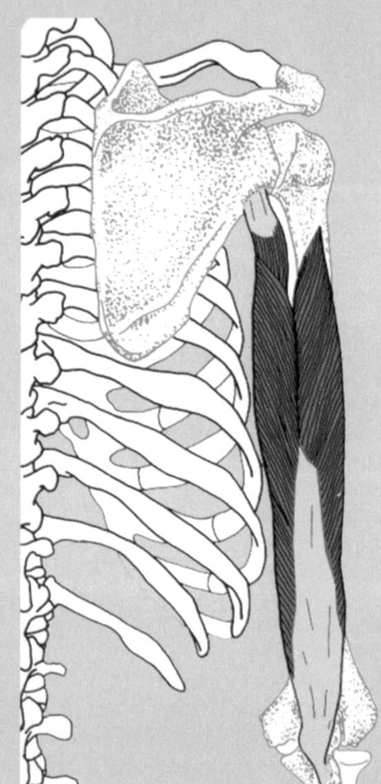

O - long - infraglenoid tubercle (Scapula)
  - lateral - lateral posterior surface of Humerus
  - medial - posterior surface of Humerus
I - olecranon (Ulna)
A - extension (elbow)
  - extension (Scapula)
NS - radial N (C6-8)
BS - deep brachial
T - extension or arm against R (in standing patient R=gravity)

Vastus Intermedius

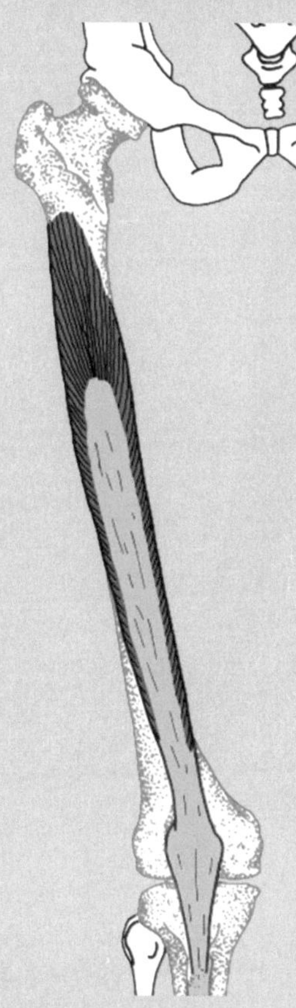

O - anterior surface of Femur
I - tibial tuberosity
A - extension (knee)
NS - femoral N (L2-4)
BS - femoral, lateral femoral circumflex
T - extension of knee in sitting patient
BS - ulnar
T - ability to extend the knee in the sitting patient

Vastus Lateralis

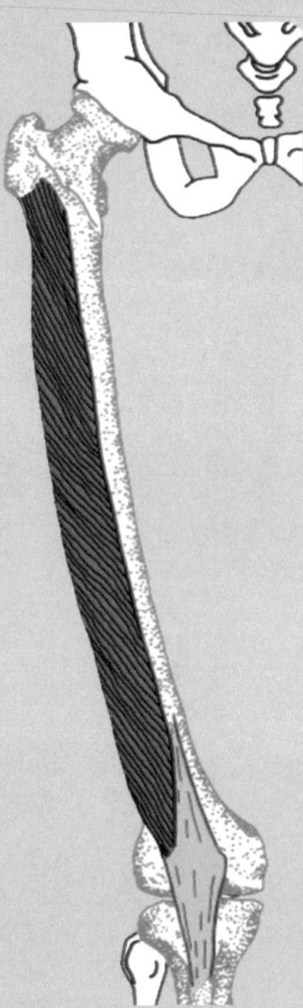

O - lateral lip of linea aspera (Femur)
I - tibial tuberosity
A - extension (knee)
NS - femoral N (L2-4)
BS - femoral, lateral femoral circumflex
T - extension of knee in sitting patient

Vastus Medialis

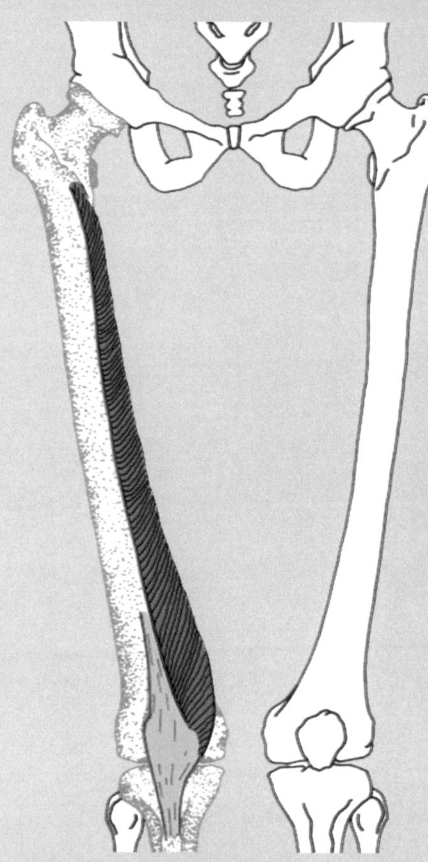

O - medial lip pf linea aspera (Femur)
I - tibial tuberosity
A - extension (knee)
NS - femoral N (L2-4)
BS - femoral
T - extension of knee in sitting patient

Zygomaticus

part of muscles of facial expression

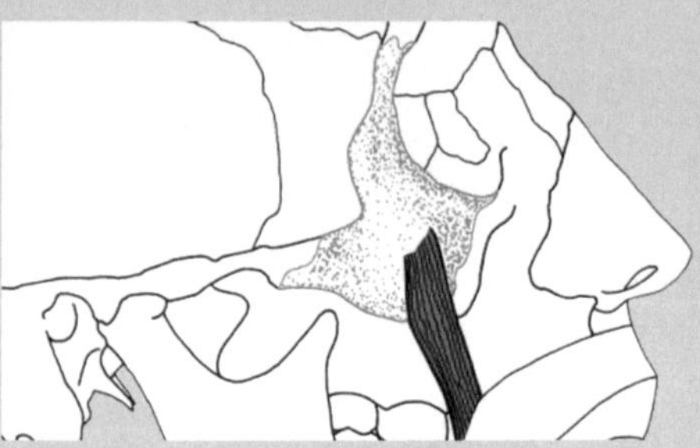

Major

O - Zygoma - cheekbone
I - deep fascia at the angle of the mouth
A - draws mouth back smiling/laughing - Major
NS - facial N (CNV)
BS - facial
T - smile

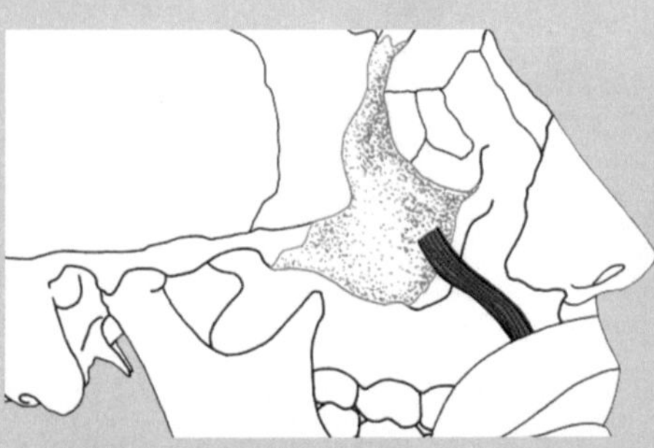

Minor

O - Zygoma – cheekbone
- deep fascia of the upper lip
A - maintains nasolabial furrow - philtum
NS - facial N (CNV)
BS - facial
often lost in cosmetic surgery i.e. no skin crease from nose to lips

Notes:

Complete your 'A to Z' set...

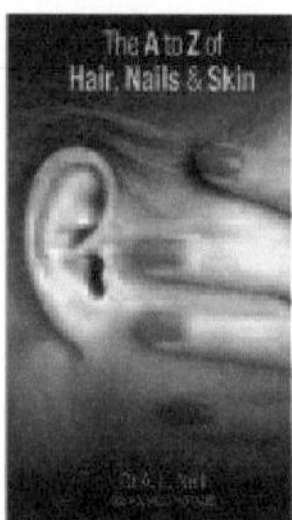

The A to Z of Hair, Nails & Skin

ISBN 978-1-921930-027

The structure of the biggest & most visible organ in the body THE SKIN, is described in detail along with its associated structures. The book has 3 distinct sections each listed in the A to Z way, with clear colourful diagrams. A large Common Terms section explains & illustrates terminology on the subject. With over 230 pages & 280 illustrations it still fits in your pocket for convenience.

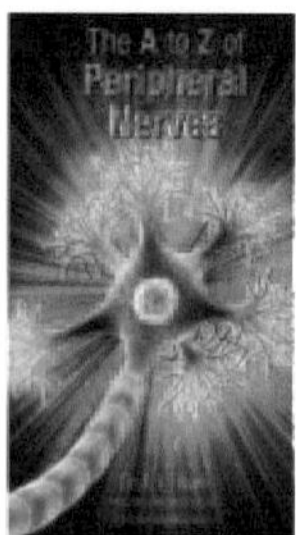

The A to Z of Peripheral Nerves

ISBN 978-1-921930-05-8

The origins, pathways, branches and functions of all the Peripheral nerves are listed alphabetically and illustrated individually. The main content includes neurological testing techniques, basic structural components of the nervous system and overviews of the major nerve plexi. It begins with a comprehensive glossary of all terms, and illustrations of basic anatomical principles. With over 230 pages and 290 illustrations this strong little book still fits in your pocket.

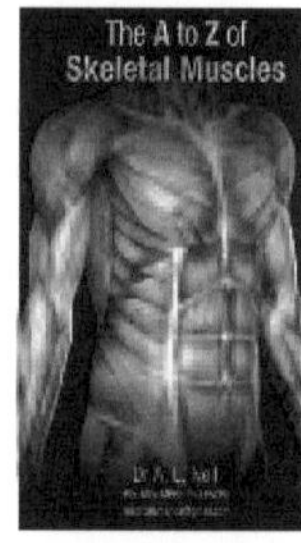

The A to Z of Skeletal Muscles

ISBN 978-1-921930-188

The origins, insertions, blood & nerve supply for all muscles are listed alphabetically with separate illustrations. All the major muscle groups, their common names their functions, along with cross-referencing and regional tagging are included. Basic structural components of the skeletal muscle system are included with a comprehensive glossary of all terms used in the field. With over 230 pages and 290 illustrations this strong little book still fits in your pocket

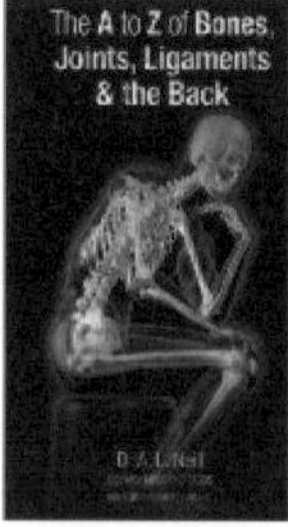

The A to Z of Bones, Joints, Ligaments & the BACK

ISBN 978-1-921930-19-5

All the bones, joints and ligaments of the body including teeth are listed alphabetically. At least 2 views of each bone and joint are illustrated. The Range of movement and basic structure of all the skeletal components are categorized and illustrated. There is a separate section on the back – Vertebral Column where it is discussed as a functioning unit. Over 260 pages and 300 illustrations make this little pocket book invaluable.

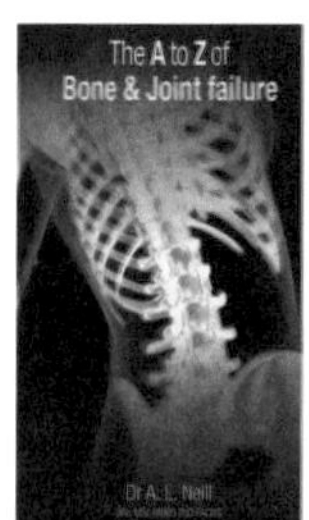

The A to Z of Bones and Joint Failure

ISBN 978-1-921930-03-4

All the bones, joints and ligaments of the body have been covered in the A to Z book on these tissues – so this is the follow-up book on their pathology analysing their failures due to various causes. It goes into the microstructure, development, control and formation and how these tissues interact and change under stress and with age. There are over 280 pages and 350 illustrations in this concise pocket book reference.

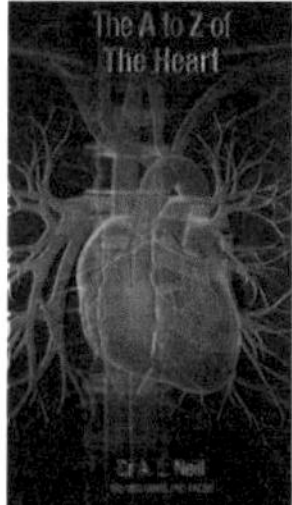

The A to Z of the Heart

ISBN 978-1-921930-16-4

The heart is comprehensively illustrated along with the great vessels. This book also includes illustrations of all the major vascular structures and describes the circulation of the major organs and systems. The clinical section contains examination and testing of the heart and blood vessel flow. Arteries, veins, capillaries and lymphatics their pathways and special features are present in this book of over 240 pages and 300 illustrations.

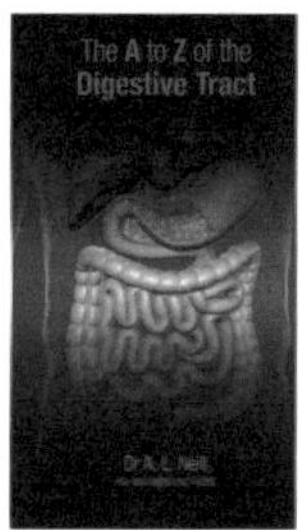

The A to Z of the Digestive Tract

ISBN 978-1-921930-00-3

The Digestive tract is one long tunnel from food to faeces – its components are individually illustrated, colour tagged and listed alphabetically along with many of its adjunct organs. Their structure and functions are also clearly described along with sectional overviews. In particular detailed descriptions of the intricacies of the oral cavity, the processes of swallowing are included in this book of 240 pages and 300 illustrations.

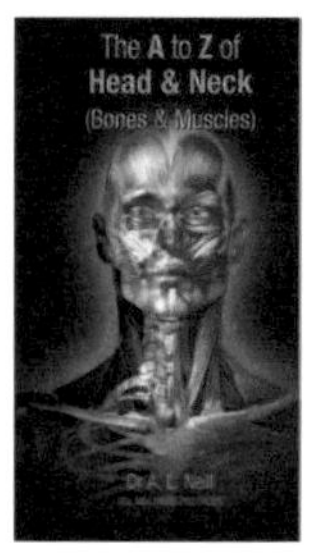

The A to Z of the Head and Neck Muscles & Bones

ISBN 978-1-921930-12-6

interactions between the many muscular layers of this area, listing alphabetically and illustrating each muscle individually in one section – then examining the individual bones and teeth in the same manner. The skull is also illustrated as a unit, in this book of 280 pages and 300 illustrations.